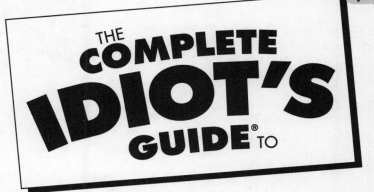

THE COMPLETE IDIOT'S GUIDE TO

Better Skin

by Lucy Beale and Angela Jensen

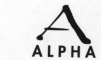

ALPHA

A member of Penguin Group (USA) Inc.

To my sister, Marcie, for her courage and love.—Lucy

To my son, Lukas, for all his patience and to my sister, Paula,
for her encouragement and for always being there for me.—Angela

ALPHA BOOKS

Published by the Penguin Group

Penguin Group (USA) Inc., 375 Hudson Street, New York, New York 10014, U.S.A.

Penguin Group (Canada), 10 Alcorn Avenue, Toronto, Ontario, Canada M4V 3B2 (a division of Pearson Penguin Canada Inc.)

Penguin Books Ltd, 80 Strand, London WC2R 0RL, England

Penguin Ireland, 25 St Stephen's Green, Dublin 2, Ireland (a division of Penguin Books Ltd)

Penguin Group (Australia), 250 Camberwell Road, Camberwell, Victoria 3124, Australia (a division of Pearson Australia Group Pty Ltd)

Penguin Books India Pvt Ltd, 11 Community Centre, Panchsheel Park, New Delhi —110 017, India

Penguin Group (NZ), cnr Airborne and Rosedale Roads, Albany, Auckland 1310, New Zealand (a division of Pearson New Zealand Ltd)

Penguin Books (South Africa) (Pty) Ltd, 24 Sturdee Avenue, Rosebank, Johannesburg 2196, South Africa

Penguin Books Ltd, Registered Offices: 80 Strand, London WC2R 0RL, England

International Standard Book Number: 1-59257-286-3
Library of Congress Catalog Card Number: 2004111437

06 05 04   8 7 6 5 4 3 2 1

Interpretation of the printing code: The rightmost number of the first series of numbers is the year of the book's printing; the rightmost number of the second series of numbers is the number of the book's printing. For example, a printing code of 04-1 shows that the first printing occurred in 2004.

Printed in the United States of America

Note: This publication contains the opinions and ideas of its authors. It is intended to provide helpful and informative material on the subject matter covered. It is sold with the understanding that the authors and publisher are not engaged in rendering professional services in the book. If the reader requires personal assistance or advice, a competent professional should be consulted.

The authors and publisher specifically disclaim any responsibility for any liability, loss, or risk, personal or otherwise, which is incurred as a consequence, directly or indirectly, of the use and application of any of the contents of this book.

Most Alpha books are available at special quantity discounts for bulk purchases for sales promotions, premiums, fundraising, or educational use. Special books, or book excerpts, can also be created to fit specific needs.

For details, write: Special Markets, Alpha Books, 375 Hudson Street, New York, NY 10014.

Publisher: *Marie Butler-Knight*
Product Manager: *Phil Kitchel*
Senior Managing Editor: *Jennifer Chisholm*
Senior Acquisitions Editor: *Renee Wilmeth*
Development Editor: *Nancy D. Lewis*
Production Editor: *Janette Lynn*

Copy Editor: *Amy Borrelli*
Cartoonist: *Shannon Wheeler*
Cover/Book Designer: *Trina Wurst*
Indexer: *Heather McNeil*
Layout: *Ayanna Lacey*
Proofreading: *Mary Hunt*

Contents at a Glance

Contents

Foreword

Treating skin with ease in today's world couldn't be more complex. However, the authors of *The Complete Idiot's Guide to Better Skin* have put together an effortless approach that's twenty-first century savvy. They will guide you with clarity through the basics of skin care and skin health to the latest in cosmeceutical products, and even more advanced clinical options in dermatology and plastic surgery.

We proudly support this book since Cultura believes so much in the appropriate education of patients regarding skin care, and we have set ourselves apart from others by teaching the Cultura Integrated Approach. Every patient should understand the principles and strategy of short and long term skin treatments and be involved in a comprehensive program that integrates their home skin care regimen with their aesthetic spa therapy and targeted medical and surgical treatments, when required. We are pleased to see a book that acts like an encyclopedia for great skin health providing valuable knowledge in the ever-changing cosmetic therapy industry.

This guide by Lucy Beale and Angela Jensen will get you started with good habits and takes you beyond skin care to address new approaches in clinical treatments, nutrition, and aging. Get ready to unveil beautiful skin!

Eliot F. Battle Jr., MD
Cosmetic Dermatologist and Laser Surgeon, Cultura's co-founder

Monte O. Harris, MD
Facial Plastic and Reconstructive Surgeon, Cultura's co-founder

Dawn M. Espinoza
Aesthetician and Director of Education at Cultura

Introduction

Yes, you can have great skin that's radiant, plump, and moist. By taking excellent care of your skin on a day-to-day basis, you can enjoy the rewards of beautiful skin every day of your life.

It's never too late to get started. So whether you're in your 20s or in your 70s, whether you're a man or a woman, start today by discovering your skin type and creating a daily skin care ritual.

Approach your skin and face with love and a positive attitude. And patience. Learn the basics of good skin care. Develop new habits that work for your skin type. With a little work, you'll have the beautiful skin you've always wanted, and you'll be able to maintain it for life.

How This Book Is Organized

This book is divided into seven parts:

Part 1, "All About Skin," tells you what skin is, what it's composed of, and about skin cell functions. You'll learn about the dermis and epidermis and the many layers of the skin. As you age, so does your skin. You'll learn what your skin needs in each decade of life.

Part 2, "Basic Skin Care Routines," presents you with a questionnaire to determine your genetic skin type. You'll learn the daily skin care ritual that works for your skin type. Choose from chemical, enzyme, or mechanical exfoliation techniques to increase skin cell turnover rate. You'll learn the best hair-removal techniques and discover the secrets to a close and tidy shave—for both men and women. Treatments for eyes, neck, and lips are included.

Part 3, "At the Store: Cosmeceuticals and Skin Care Products," gives you inside information on skin care products. You'll learn which ingredients, including cosmeceuticals, to use on your skin. You'll learn the differences between the expensive and the discount store brands—which are often minimal. If you prefer to add a touch of color or foundation, we'll tell you how to choose products for your skin type and how to apply them.

Part 4, "Combating Common Skin Conditions," shows you how to correct temporary skin conditions such as acne, congestion, blemishes, rosacea, dehydration, sun damage, abnormal pigmentation, premature aging, and menopausal skin. The good news is that all these conditions can be corrected and healed.

Part 5, "Creating Healthy Skin Through a Healthy Lifestyle," teaches you a lifestyle program that benefits your skin from the inside out and gives you a radiant glow. Learn about water, diet, and the environment. Detoxify your body to keep your skin clear and exercise to eliminate double chins and maintain muscle tone.

Part 6, "Home Treatments for Your Skin," clues you in to the newest fads for improving the appearance of your skin at home. Do machines offered on infomercials really work? We'll give you the lowdown. One system that's moved beyond fad status is facial exercises, and you can get started right away with the exercises in this section.

Part 7, "Professional Treatments," gives you all the information you need to make wise choices concerning treatments by skin care professionals, including dermatologists, plastic surgeons, paramedical estheticians, and skin care technicians.

Skin Care Bulletins

The sidebars in this book offer techniques, tips, and warnings that guide you to achieving better skin.

Clarifying Words

Definitions of words and concepts that increase your understanding of your skin and good skin care.

Skin-spiration

Tips to inspire you and advise you about skin care techniques.

Wrinkle Guard

Warnings that help you avoid mistakes in caring for your skin.

Body of Knowledge

Good information about many aspects of skin and skin care.

Acknowledgments

Lucy warmly gives thanks to her co-author, Angela Jensen, for her dedication and hard work in sharing her expertise; to Kathleen Dreier for introducing her to Angela; to Patrick Partridge Jr., her stepson, who valiantly reviewed the manuscript and made style and grammar suggestions; to Linda Chae and Clara Mueller for sharing their expertise; and to Pamela Hill of Facial Aesthetics, for her detailed and helpful technical review.

Lucy gives a loving thank-you to her husband, Patrick, for his encouragement and support. Lucy thanks her literary agent, Marilyn Allen, for her persistent work in making this book a reality.

Lucy and Angela thank the staff at Alpha Books, including their editor, Renee Wilmeth, for believing so strongly in the success of this project, and Nancy Lewis, development editor.

Angela acknowledges Judy Thealand, her inspiration and teacher in the field of esthetics; Kathleen Dreier, who connected her with this opportunity to share her knowledge; Lucy Beale, who believed in her and had confidence in her expertise; and to her mother, Judy, who instilled in her the courage to take on new projects and challenges.

Special Thanks to the Technical Reviewer

The Complete Idiot's Guide to Better Skin was reviewed by an expert who double-checked the accuracy of what you'll learn here, to help us ensure that this book gives you everything you need to know about better skin. Special thanks are extended to Pamela Hill.

Trademarks

All terms mentioned in this book that are known to be or are suspected of being trademarks or service marks have been appropriately capitalized. Alpha Books and Penguin Group (USA) Inc. cannot attest to the accuracy of this information. Use of a term in this book should not be regarded as affecting the validity of any trademark or service mark.

Part 1

All About Skin

Your skin is a fabulously complex biological organ—in fact, it's the largest organ in your body. Every aspect of your life is reflected in your skin. Oh, the tales your skin could tell. Actually, it already does. It tells everyone about your lifestyle and the general state of your health.

In this part of the book, you'll learn how your skin functions and exactly how it reflects your inner health, and even your inner thoughts. Then, you'll track the changes skin goes through as we age decade by decade, from childhood through your 60s and 70s. Usually, people in their 20s are thought to have the most ideal skin, but you'll see that at any age you can have better skin, provided you start now to develop the best skin care habits.

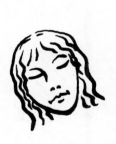 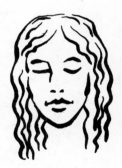 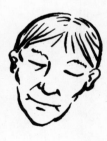

Your Amazing Skin

In This Chapter

- Why your skin is important
- Setting a goal for great skin
- Caring for skin with serenity and love
- The anatomy of skin

There's a reason that skin care is a $40 billion–a-year industry. There's a reason that beauty parlors and salons are everywhere, why entire aisles of grocery stores and entire sections of department stores are dedicated to skin care, and why plenty of advertising is devoted to skin care products. It's the same reason you're holding this book: The state of your skin matters to you.

Your skin is your constant representative to the world at large. It's often the first thing about you that a stranger sees, and your skin speaks for you in every social situation. For better or for worse, others judge you by the appearance of your skin, and like it or not, you do the same. It's a fundamental part of how we size one another up.

For the entire course of human history, ever since we made our homes in caves, our primitive instinct has been to select a healthy partner when searching for a mate. This ensures the healthy continuance of future generations. Prospective mates would be wary of a person with smallpox scars, rashes, and other skin problems that could signal disease. Skin condition isn't superficial; it's an indication of our overall physical health.

In today's world, the quest for better skin continues. In a sense, survival is still at stake. We want to attract the best partner, the best job, the best friends, and the best clients. Having clear, healthy skin is a part of how we go about making those things happen. Essentially, we want our outer skin to reflect our inner quality.

We ask a lot from our skin, and to achieve better skin we need to give it plenty of loving care in two basic ways. We need to pay attention to what we put on our skin, and we need to pay attention to what we put inside ourselves. As you'll learn throughout this book, what you put inside your body is just as important as what you apply topically to your skin. But when you take good care both inside and out, you can have the great skin you've always wanted.

In this chapter, you'll learn all about your skin—what it is and how it works. Once you understand what your skin is made of and how it functions, you'll be able to develop a skin care routine based on good science and personal insight.

The Goal of Better Skin

Great skin is a status symbol. It's a reflection of health and well-being, youthfulness and vitality. Having great skin once meant having the time and the money to seek perfection. Today, with a little effort anyone can have great skin.

More than just time and money, having better skin means doing what works—daily skin care coupled with living a healthy lifestyle. Excellent skin care products are available in every price range. You can purchase high-quality cosmetic and *cosmeceutical* skin care products on a shoestring budget from discount stores, and your skin can look just as good as that of a person who spends hundreds of dollars a month.

Clarifying Words

A **cosmeceutical** is a bioactive skin care ingredient that actually alters the skin and its underlying health. Cosmeceuticals are often combined with cosmetic ingredients in skin care products. DMAE and green tea are examples of cosmeceuticals.

You're on a quest to have better skin, but just what is that? Most people could claim they'd know great skin if they saw it, and certainly you know when your own skin looks good and when it doesn't, but let's get specific. How do we define great skin?

First of all, great skin simply looks good. The skin is plump and radiant, with even pigmentation. The skin glows just slightly with a dewy moisture, rather than being matte and dull in appearance. The skin is elastic and has no obviously visible wrinkles or sagging.

Next, the skin has no blemishes, rashes, or redness. The skin neither flakes nor peels. The skin glows clean and clear.

Skin-spiration

Be careful not to judge your skin based on the pictures of models in advertisements or publicity shots of movie stars in magazines. The models' photos have been airbrushed to erase pores and tiny wrinkles around the eyes and mouth. Actresses on the red carpet have undergone intense facials and skin treatments, and can only present perfect skin to the photographers with the assistance of top-paid makeup artists. You have no way of knowing how their skin actually looks in person or in their everyday life.

Now, let's get real. The definition of great skin simply doesn't occur spontaneously. Having better skin takes work, it requires making lifestyle changes, and, quite honestly, it requires making lifestyle sacrifices.

Even the best skin moves in and out of greatness. Everyone should expect the occasional blemish or phase of dull-looking skin. These things are caused by hormonal changes, late nights, stress, and just plain living life. But you can learn to remedy those conditions quickly, and you can learn how to prepare your skin for those big events when it's even more important for your skin to radiate and glow.

All skin ages, though with proper maintenance and care, you can hold back the ravages of time and present a youthful-looking visage at any age.

Better skin is a goal, and it's within your reach. The more carefully and lovingly you pursue the goal, the higher your reward—lovely and radiant skin.

Loving Your Skin

As you work toward creating better skin, your attitude will make a big difference in your results. Approach your skin with love and appreciation regardless of its current condition. Even if you think your skin is a mess right now, it won't get better unless you approach it with love.

Love and appreciation mean gentleness, patience, and generosity. It also means using valid scientific knowledge and treatments to improve your skin. Add to that serenity—the serenity that comes from knowing that the more you love and appreciate your skin and face, the more your skin will come into balance and perform as you desire. Stress plays a major factor in skin conditions such as breakouts and *congestion*, so relax now and you'll soon see the positive results in your skin.

If you approach your skin with a sense of urgency, frustration, and anger, you will increase your stress levels. An increase in stress triggers production of the stress hormone, *cortisol*. Cortisol causes inflammation in the body and on your skin. Inflamed skin means more eruptions, more wrinkles, more sagging—you get the picture. If you approach your skin with negative emotions, guess what? You make the situation worse.

Skin-spiration

Beauty is far more than skin deep. What you put on the surface of your skin is only one part. Other parts include what you eat and how you live. Add to that your attitude about life, yourself, and your skin and you have the complete package that affects your skin.

Clarifying Words

Congested skin is skin that's bumpy and stopped up. The natural oils and skin sloughing has slowed down, leaving the skin looking unclear and dull. **Cortisol** is an adrenal-cortex hormone. Any type of physical or mental stress induces the release of cortisol. Too much ongoing cortisol in the body causes inflammation and irritation. It's thought to be a cause of chronic disease conditions such as diabetes, heart disease, and autoimmune disorders.

Skin—the Body's Wonder Organ

The skin that covers your body is a highly complex and durable organ. In fact, it's the largest organ of the body. Biologically, skin serves many purposes.

◆ The skin protects the internal organs from sun damage and other insults (although you need to use sunscreen to assist the skin with this function), it helps regulate body temperature, and it provides the first barrier of immune system defense against bacterias, viruses, pollution, and toxic chemicals.

◆ The skin excretes bodily waste products. Some are excreted through *sebum;* some are excreted through breakouts and eruptions.

- The skin sweats to cool the body's core temperature. In the process, it cools the body. Sweat also carries toxins from the body.

- The skin absorbs radiation from the sun, which helps regulate the hormonal system and your sleeping and waking circadian rhythms.

- The skin also works with sunlight to produce the necessary nutrient vitamin D on the surface of your skin. Vitamin D is a necessary nutrient for bones, skin, teeth, and many metabolic processes.

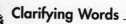

Clarifying Words

Sebum is the semifluid secretion of the sebaceous glands, consisting chiefly of fat, keratin, and cellular material. **Antioxidants** are chemicals that neutralize free radicals that cause damage to the body and skin. These come from eating fruits and vegetables and also can be applied topically to help heal the surface of the skin.

- The skin produces melanin, the coloring of your skin. Melanin helps protect the body from sun damage, and gives your skin tone. The amount of melanin in your skin is determined by your genetics.

Between one half and two thirds of your total blood supply is always circulating through the skin. The blood nourishes the skin with vitamins, minerals, *antioxidants*, and other important nutrients.

Within the layers of your skin is a large portion of your body's lymph supply. The lymph system carries toxins away from the vital organs of the body and sends them on to be excreted. Lymph fluid is clear and is very close to the surface of the skin. In Chapter 23, you'll learn how to get the lymph fluid moving to keep your skin clear and soft.

Your skin does all this work by itself—after all, that's its job. But you can help it out. You can actually assist your skin in doing its job, and when you do, you'll have better-looking skin. The harder your skin has to work on its own without the benefits of your daily skin care rituals and healing salon and medical treatments, the faster it ages and the more worn-out it looks.

Throughout this book, and especially in Part 5, you'll find plenty of suggestions for supporting

Body of Knowledge

The mathematical facts of skin are truly incredible. Each square inch of skin on a normal-size body contains 65 hairs, 90 to 100 sebaceous glands, 650 sweat glands and 9,500,000 skin cells, plus 19 yards of blood vessels and 19,500 sensory cells.

your skin. Some of them you may already do, such as wearing protective sunscreen and drinking plenty of purified water. Others you might not have even heard of. But the more you do to aid your skin in its work, the happier you'll be with how it looks.

The Anatomy of Your Skin

As you read through this book, you'll find references to the various biological parts of the skin. Each part serves an important function in your overall health. When each part functions correctly, your skin looks great.

The Universal Skin Diagram.

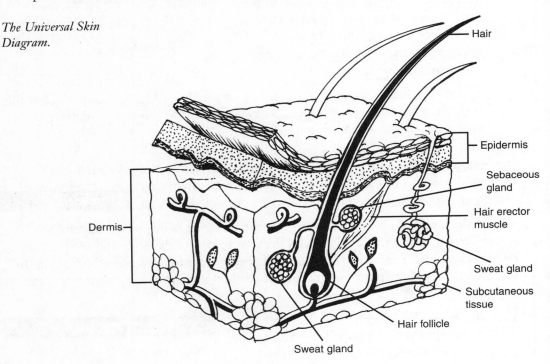

Epidermis

The epidermis is the top layer of skin—the part you see. Within that top layer are six sublayers, each with a special function. The epidermis is between 0.5 to 1.0 millimeters thick. The use of both cosmetics and cosmeceuticals affects the epidermis, although cosmeceuticals penetrate beyond the epidermis. Three major types of cells make up the epidermis: keratinocytes, melanocytes, and Langerhans cells. The condition of your epidermis determines how "fresh" your skin looks and how well your skin absorbs and holds moisture from outside sources.

At the deepest part of the epidermis, the stratum germinativum, also called the stratum basal are immature, rapidly dividing keratinocytes that make the protein keratin. As they mature, keratinocytes lose water, flatten out, and move upward. Eventually, at the end of their life cycle, they reach the top layer of the epidermis, called the stratum disjunctum.

The stratum disjunctum is a protective crust consisting mainly of dead keratinocytes, hardened proteins (keratins), and lipids. The dead cells continuously slough off and are replaced by new ones from below in a process that completely renews itself every three to five weeks. *Exfoliants*, such as peels and scrubs, remove the dead skin cells, keratins, and lipids, thus speeding up skin renewal.

Clarifying Words

Exfoliants are skin care products that break down and remove keratinized cells (dead skin cells that build up and cover up the newer skin underneath). Even skin functioning at peak performance and normal skin can benefit from an exfoliant. Exfoliants help restore that healthy, translucent glow we all strive for.

The second layer from the surface is the stratum corneum. When cells reach this level, traveling from inside out, they are nearing the final stages of life. No water from inside the body reaches this layer, but water from outside the skin can. Certain lipids, fats, and oils make up the natural moisturizing factor (NMF) found in the stratum corneum. The cells here are densely packed and slough off when exfoliated. NMF is simulated in cosmetics because NMF can absorb moisture from the air and from skin care products.

Body of Knowledge

Skin is thinnest on the eyelids and thickest on the palms of the hands and soles of the feet.

The third layer is only found on the palms and soles of the feet. Called the stratum lucidum, it comprises translucent cells filled with densely packed filaments. This layer gives your palms and soles extra padding.

The fourth layer of the epidermis is the stratum granulosum. The cells here look like distinct granules made up of keratin protein. This layer also contains NMF.

The fifth layer is the stratum spinosum. The Langerhans cells are found in this layer. A part of the immune system that prevent foreign substances from penetrating the skin, allergic responses occur in this layer as the Langerhans cells do their job. Squamous cell carcinomas, or skin cancers, originate in this layer of the epidermis as well.

The sixth layer, the stratum germinativum, is where the keratinocytes are formed and where they begin their journey to the outer layer of the epidermis. Melanocytes, the cells that produce melanin, also originate at this level, as well as basal cell carcinomas, a different form of skin cancer.

Dermis

The dermis is beneath the epidermis and maintains the structure of the skin. It contains the sweat glands, *sebaceous glands*, hair follicles, lymphatic vessels that contain lymphatic fluid, and blood vessels. It's thicker than the epidermis and is composed of a mesh of collagen and elastin fibers.

Collagen and *elastin* are proteins. Collagen provides structural support; elastin gives the skin resilience. Fibroblasts are the cells that synthesize collagen and elastin. They need to function properly for skin to hold its shape and look youthful.

Sweat, uric acid, and sebum reach the top surface of the epidermis through pore openings. This mixture gives skin its slightly acidic protective mantle which protects the skin from bacteria and debris. The protective mantle is commonly referred to as the acid mantle.

Clarifying Words

Sebaceous glands produce sebum—an oily substance that lubricates and waterproofs the skin. Too little sebum results in dry skin; overproduction leads to oily skin and acne. **Collagen** is a protein forming the chief constituent of the connective tissues and bones. It gives skin strength and durability. Age-related declines in collagen production cause thinning of the skin, wrinkles, and sagging. Vitamin C and eating foods rich in amino acids stimulate collagen production. **Elastin** helps maintain skin resilience and elasticity. When elastin is abundant and undamaged, the skin regains its shape after being folded or stretched.

Subcutaneous Layer

Underneath it all is the subcutaneous layer of the skin. This layer contains adipose tissue, or fat tissue, which serves as a shock absorber and heat insulator, protecting the body from cold and outside trauma.

The subcutaneous fat lies on the muscles that cover the bones. The whole skin structure is attached by connective tissues. The attachment is quite loose, so the skin can move fairly freely. As a person ages, subcutaneous tissue is lost, leading to sagging and wrinkles.

Skin care products and other skin care treatments don't directly affect or rebuild the subcutaneous skin layer.

The Least You Need to Know

- Clear, glowing skin is within your reach through careful skin care techniques and living a healthy lifestyle.

- Be gentle with your skin in both your actions and thoughts to keep it—and you—calm, soothed, and serene by preventing inflammation.

- The skin is amazing in its complexity and function.

- Understanding how skin functions will give you the knowledge you need to have great-looking skin.

Caring for Skin at Every Age

In This Chapter

◆ Understanding how skin changes with age

◆ Specific skin care for every decade of life

◆ Establishing good lifetime skin care habits

◆ Treatments and techniques by age

Better skin is attainable at any age for both men and women. However, the criteria for great skin shifts as a person gets chronologically older. In each decade, your skin has certain characteristics and will face certain challenges—pun intended.

For example, in the teenage years, skin is plump, dewy, and moist with no visible wrinkles or sagging. However, increasing hormonal production brings with it more oil production, leading to breakouts and acne. Great skin as a teenager includes no visible breakouts and no suntan. As hormone production levels out with age, the oil production lessens and different challenges arise.

By mastering the challenges of skin care for each decade, you can attain better skin for each age of your skin. In this chapter, you'll learn what to expect from your skin at every phase of life and what to do today to ensure great skin for the rest of your life.

Skin Aging Factors

Each decade of life brings changes to your skin in two ways, intrinsic and extrinsic. *Intrinsic* changes are determined by your genetics. Just as the color of your skin, eyes, and hair are preset by your own inherited DNA, so too how your skin ages is in part determined by your DNA.

Some people are graced with fabulous skin genes, and your skin could look young well into your 50s and 60s. Other people are born with skin that wrinkles and sags earlier. While you can't do anything about your inborn genetic patterns, later in life, you can avail yourself of a wide variety of scientific and medical solutions to sagging and wrinkles.

In the next chapter, you'll use a survey to determine the genetic predisposition of your skin. You'll use this information to design a skin care program for yourself so that you can make the most of the skin you were born with.

You are in control of most *extrinsic* aging factors. They're caused by the environment and by how you care for your skin. Sun damage can be avoided by using sunscreen. Your daily maintenance rituals of cleansing, toning, and moisturizing, or lack of them will make a difference. So will keeping your hands away from breakouts and blackheads. Even avoiding frowning and grimacing can help you control extrinsic factors.

As you read about skin at each decade of life, keep in mind that you are learning the general ways that skin changes and ages, and that both your DNA and your skin care rituals can make a big difference in the quality of your skin.

Clarifying Words

Intrinsic factors are caused by your biological and genetic makeup. You were born with a certain type of skin and your DNA determines in part how it ages, your skin tone, and it's overall plumpness and glow. **Extrinsic** factors that affect skin are caused by the environment, your health, and how you treat your skin. For the most part, you can control the extrinsic factors that affect the condition of your skin.

The First Decade of Life: Infant Through Ten Years

Healthy baby skin always seems so perfect—soft, plump, dewy, and moist with plenty of fat cells to keep it pliant and full. The body's collagen and elastin are at optimal levels. The skin is superbly resilient. Scrapes and bruises seem to repair themselves overnight.

A young child's skin only needs to be washed once daily with a gentle soap to maintain its lovely texture. However, as babies turn into toddlers and then into preschoolers, inevitably children learn that making messes can be fun. They play with food, playground dirt, and their art projects. Thankfully, their faces can withstand many washings a day based on necessity.

Because children's skins are brand new, children's skin cells turn over and renew themselves naturally every 21 to 28 days.

If a child is ill with a disease such as asthma, his or her skin can show signs of stress, but the skin still has the ability to recover quickly as the illness subsides.

In these early years, do all you can to encourage good skin care habits. Make regular body movement and exercise a natural part of your child's daily routine. Face washing becomes an essential part of your child's daily self-care process, equally as important as brushing teeth and bathing.

The most important aspect of skin care in this decade is sun protection. Apply sun protection whenever your child goes outside. Make applying sunscreen non-negotiable. It's essential to the continued health of your child.

Now is the time to provide healthy, nutrient-dense foods for your child. Avoid serving junk foods and instead feed your child vegetables and fruits filled with vitamins, minerals, and antioxidants. Make sure your child eats nutritious foods at school, with friends, and at home as a way to ensure his or her overall health and well-being, and as a way to set the stage for good skin in later years. Healthy eating habits established early in life will be the good habits of the future.

CAUTION   **Wrinkle Guard** _____

Even just one serious sunburn early in life can create skin cancer 20 to 30 years later. Medical specialists now think that many adult skin cancers are the result of a lack of sun protection as children. Be sure to use an SFP15 or higher, on your children every day. Choose a sunscreen or sunblock designed for children that protects against both UVA and UVB sun radiation.

The Teenage Years: Ten to Twenty

Seemingly without warning, skin starts changing and keeps on changing throughout the teenage years. The soft, baby-type skin of youth typically faces its first challenges in this phase of life.

Two definite challenges emerge in this period. The first is the result of increased hormone production as the teenager moves through puberty. The second challenge is a teenager's desire to have better skin through acute peer pressure.

Hormonal changes signal the beginnings of adulthood. The skin has matured enough to give evidence of its genetic skin type (see the survey in Chapter 3 for more information on genetic skin types). As hormones change, the skin produces more oil due to overactive sebaceous glands, and breakouts occur. If a teenager was born with oily-type skin, his or her skin produces even more oil than other skin types, increasing the chance of breakouts. Acne-type skin develops acne that can range from slight to highly active.

The operative phrase for the teenage years is "no picking." The temptation to pick at breakouts and pimples is alluring. However, the risks are serious and include spreading the breakout to other areas of the face and inflicting harm that results in permanent scarring.

Now is the time to find reliable and effective skin care products and establish a routine of using them twice a day for cleansing, toning, and moisturizing. The skin cells are still renewing themselves every 21 to 28 days, which is ideal. Exfoliate between one to three times a week, based on skin type and frequency of breakouts. Use salicylic acid exfoliants for breakouts and acne-type skin because they have anti-bacterial qualities and go inside the pores to control bacteria. Be sure not to overdo exfoliation, as this causes inflammation, which results in more breakouts and even premature aging.

Be faithful to your skin care ritual and be sure not to overdo it, meaning don't cleanse, tone, and moisturize more than two times a day. On the other hand, make sure to follow your ritual faithfully in the morning and the evening. Never go to bed without washing your face, and never go to bed without removing makeup. During sleep is when your skin renews itself and releases waste products and toxins. This process gets backed up when you don't remove makeup and wash your face before bed and can cause congestion and dull skin.

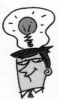

Skin-spiration

The best time to learn about skin care is in the teenage years. Teenagers care how they look and the correct education can make a difference in the quality of their skin now and throughout their lives. They can learn to avoid picking at eruptions, which creates lifelong scarring. Teenagers must use sun protection to avoid sagging, wrinkles, and dark pigmentation problems later in life.

Avoid sunbathing or tanning booths in search of the perfect tan. There's no such thing. Tanning ruins the internal structure of your skin. Sure, the tan may seem gorgeous at the moment, but it won't in 20 years when the external signs of sun damage are written all over your face in wrinkles, cross-hatched lines, and sagging skin. Cross-hatched lines go in many directions at once, making the skin's texture appear to look like dried fruit. Stay pale; stay true to your skin tone. Be proud of your natural skin color.

Use sunscreen or *sunblock* whenever you are outside. Reapply often at the beach, or whenever you are outdoors for longer than an hour or after you swim or sweat. You can't really overdo sunscreen. Make it a fact of life, and be sure to apply plenty so you protect your skin and don't tan or burn.

Clarifying Words

The FDA only recognizes the term sunscreen and not **sunblock**. Common usage of the term sunblock refers to sunscreens that use a physical barrier to reflect the sun's damaging rays off of the skin. Two sunblock ingredients are zinc oxide and titanium dioxide. Other sunscreens use a chemical barrier to prevent sunburn.

Learn how to eat nutrient-dense foods. Avoid junk foods, highly processed foods, and sugar-laden foods. Instead, choose vegetables, fruits, nuts, seeds, meats, fish, and poultry. Learn all about low-glycemic foods and make them the mainstay of your meals (see Chapter 21 for more information on low-glycemic foods). High-glycemic foods create inflammation, which shows up as breakouts and aging on the skin.

Find ways to hang out with your friends and have a good time without eating the junk foods that can cause skin inflammation. Make regular exercise an important part of your life. Participate in sports or exercise with friends by doing both aerobics and strength training.

For unusual skin problems, visit your dermatologist. Be cautious about using antibiotics, as overuse could create yeast overgrowth problems and antibiotic resistance.

Skin-spiration

In the teenage years, it's an enormous temptation to get a suntan. Glamour articles and photographs show alluringly tanned bodies in swimsuits that entice young men and women to think that having a luscious tan is a certain path to popularity and acceptance. What we know for certain is that tanning is a sure path to sun-damaged skin, wrinkles, sagging, and skin cancers. It's time to make untanned faces and bodies desirable once again. Flaunt your normal skin tone, your sun hat, and your sunscreen. If you feel you must have a tan, use sunless tanning products or face bronzers rather than sit outside in the sun.

For teenage boys, shaving becomes a daily ritual. Likewise, teenage girls are frequently removing body hair. Shaving is a great exfoliator and can help teenage skin look great. To learn how to shave properly see Chapter 6 for details.

In Your Twenties

Most people have balanced hormones by the age of 20 (however, pregnancy can play havoc with your skin). By your 20s, your hormones have settled down. Your skin typically needs minimal care for great results. Skin in good condition is dewy, moist, and radiant with no wrinkles or sagging. You may notice a couple of lines around your eyes when you squint, but those aren't really considered wrinkles.

Your skin's oil production has slowed down and your skin is starting to change. The cell renewal cycle of 21 to 28 days is also starting to slow down. If you've had acne outbreaks as a teenager, they have probably slowed down as well. Your skin still has ample amounts of collagen and elastin. Twenty-year-old skin is the benchmark of great skin for women of all ages. Enjoy your skin now and start adopting a lifestyle that will keep your skin healthy and glowing for the rest of your life.

By your early 20s, at the latest by age 25, you need to be on a daily skin care ritual of cleansing, toning, and moisturizing twice a day. Never go to sleep in your makeup.

Exfoliation becomes essential to keep your skin cells turning over quickly. Use an alpha-hydroxy (AHA) or beta-hydroxy (BHA) acid exfoliant once a month, or more often if skin is congested. You'll learn more about exfoliation in Chapter 5. The idea is to avoid the harsher exfoliants, such as glycolic acid peels or microdermabrasion, as your skin doesn't need them yet. Lactic acid is a mild exfoliant and you can use this more frequently. Otherwise, alternate AHAs or BHAs with scrubs and enzyme exfoliants, doing about one treatment per week.

Be sure to apply sunscreen every morning immediately after your skin care ritual. Reapply often if you are outdoors during the day. Keep your skin's natural color—don't even think about getting a natural suntan, and don't go near a tanning booth. If you have spent time in the sun with unprotected skin, your skin could start showing sun damage in your 20s.

To keep your skin healthy, schedule regular exercise into your daily agenda. Exercise vigorously at least three times a week. Do aerobic, strength, and flexibility training. Take a vitamin-mineral supplement to assure that you are getting the nutrition you need to support healthy skin.

This is the decade when many women decide to start families and become pregnant. Skin changes during pregnancy, often for the better, but sometimes not. During pregnancy, skin can become congested with breakouts due to the change in hormones. Don't panic. Be very gentle with your skin. Maintain your daily skin care ritual using products designed for breakouts and congestion. Your skin will return to normal when you stop breastfeeding.

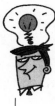

Skin-spiration

Both men and women may start gaining weight in their 20s. Take action now to eat well and exercise to master your weight and your size. Weight gain and weight loss play a large role in creating sagging skin, wrinkles, and double chins. That way, you can avoid weight gain in later years. If your pregnancy weight gain resulted in visible stretch marks, you can use one of the wonderful stretch mark creams now available at the drugstore or health-food store.

Thirty to Forty

Skin in your 30s can easily look great. True, you no longer have the skin of a 20-year-old, but your skin still looks young and vibrant, with few, if any, lines or wrinkles. Lines and wrinkles in your thirties depend on the amount of sunscreen you used or sun exposure as a young person. Your level of facial animation can also make a difference. Those with more expressive faces will have more lines. These are called "dynamic" lines. Your skin looks healthy and still has plenty of collagen and elastin. It doesn't take much for your skin to look great.

At some point in your 30s, your skin experiences a major turning point. This coincides with the time when your metabolism starts to slow down, partially because muscle mass starts to decline. Skin cell turnover is slower, perhaps even as slow as every 40 days. Your skin starts wrinkling, particularly around the eyes. Sun damage from earlier in life shows up as sagging and skin discolorations. Collagen and elastin depletion also cause the skin to begin sagging ever so slightly.

In this decade your skin shifts as it begins to age. But even with all these changes, your skin can still look fabulous. Be consistent with your skin care. Continue your daily skin ritual of cleansing, toning, and moisturizing. Now is the time to start using glycolic acid exfoliation products regularly. Start with once a week, and

Body of Knowledge

What goes in your body is more important than what goes on your skin. Great skin never just comes out of a bottle. Using the most expensive skin care products can't make up for poor nutrition, smoking, and lack of exercise or sleep.

gradually add one more treatment per week, up to two to three times a week, based on need. Glycolic acid has been shown to assist the skin in rebuilding collagen.

Consider getting a chemical peel once a month from a professional skin care specialist. At the very least, consider a professional facial and skin treatment at the change of seasons. Get checked for skin cancer by a dermatologist or medical doctor every year.

Get plenty of exercise, rest, and sleep. In your 20s, you could get away with staying out late and still looking great the next morning. In your 30s and beyond, dancing into the wee hours of the night shows up the next morning. Your face may swell and bags and dark circles could develop under your eyes.

Continual high stress levels result in inflammation, wrinkles, and sagging. When eating, choose the foods that keep your skin healthy such as low-glycemic carbohydrates, essential fatty acids, and complete protein. Avoid cortisol-inducing foods and beverages, such as coffee, caffeine, and alcoholic beverages, which can cause inflammation and irritation. See Chapter 21 for more specific food recommendations.

Forty to Fifty

Within the past 10 years, skin care for the over-40 age group has become excellent at forestalling the ravages of time. Your skin can look terrific, thanks to cosmeceuticals and a wide variety of minor medical skin procedures.

Great skin in this decade has minimal sun damage and few expression lines, although you can expect to have some lines around your eyes. The skin can still appear dewy, moist, and radiant. Oily-type skin generally has an easier time of this, as the skin produces more natural oil, but with proper moisturizing and a healthy lifestyle, any skin type can look ideal. Great skin continues to exude vitality and has an even pigmentation. .

Many men may have a new skin care concern in their 40s—a receding hairline. Care for the balding areas around your face just as you care for the rest of your facial skin. Cleanse, tone, and moisturize twice a day. Apply sunscreen faithfully every day. Yes, you should even exfoliate the balding areas.

Any serious health challenges, such as diabetes, high blood pressure, or autoimmune disorders affect the health of your skin. The skin may become more sensitive and inflamed and could be red or flushed most of the time. The skin condition rosacea could begin in this decade.

For women, the 40s usually signal the start of perimenopause. At this time, skin oil production slows, leaving skin drier, and skin may start to become thinner and more translucent.

Continue your daily skin care ritual, taking into consideration that you may need to switch products or skin care lines as your skin becomes drier and more sensitive. Start doing chemical peels once a month to encourage more rapid skin cell turnover. Exfoliate at home two to three times a week with AHAs, scrubs, or *enzymes*. Use cosmeceuticals, vitamin C, and alpha lipoic acid to help reverse the visible signs of aging.

Consider asking your dermatologist for a prescription for Retin-A or Renova to assist your skin with rejuvenation. These vitamin A–derivative products help to rebuild collagen. Use sunscreen or sunblock daily and avoid sun exposure. Check yourself for skin cancers regularly and have your dermatologist or medical doctor check as well. Refer to Chapter 16 on sun damage to learn how to check for skin changes that could indicate cancers.

You may want to consider such medical procedures as Botox or collagen injections to improve your appearance and to temporarily melt away lines and wrinkles. Laser resurfacing can destroy deep brown pigmentation and enlarged or broken capillaries.

If you haven't already, become more conscientious about your eating and exercise habits. Get plenty of aerobic exercise and strength training to boost your metabolism. Eat more foods that contain phytoestrogens. See Chapter 21 for a list of foods containing phytoestrogens.

> **Clarifying Words**
>
> **Enzymes** are food products or supplements that aid in digestion. Papaya contains the enzyme papain, and pineapple contains the enzyme bromelain. Both are commonly used as aids to the stomach to enhance digestion. These same enzymes, when used on the face, "digest" or break down dead skin cells and other cellular waste. They clear out the gunk and leave a brightened complexion.

In Your Fifties

If you've been good to yourself and your skin, by now you are enjoying the rewards. Your skin has an even skin tone, with perhaps some slightly darker pigmentation spots. If you've used sun protection regularly, your skin has enough collagen and elastin to remain plump and smooth. You may have some sagging, but not much. By your 50s, expression lines are a fact of life, especially if you have dynamic facial expressions. You can still have dewy, moist, and radiant skin, but you find that you have to work at it.

Men's skin is more robust than women's because men don't lose their reproductive capacity through menopause. Men's skin sags less because men have more vital collagen and elastin, provided they've stayed out of the sun or used good sun protection. Men need to be on the watch for errant hair growth on the eyebrows, ears, and nose.

Learn to tame your eyebrows yourself or employ the services of an expert at a salon. Be sure to check your skin, including your scalp if balding, for skin cancers.

Maintain good skin care habits by sticking to your daily skin care ritual. You can be aggressive with encouraging skin cell turnover by using glycolic peels and frequent exfoliation. If you've spent time in the sun, the damage is showing as sagging skin from collagen and elastin damage. Deep brown pigmentation spots are another result of sun damage. You can reverse some of this damage by the use of cosmeceuticals, vitamin C, and alpha lipoic acid. Both glycolic peels and Retin-A or Renova assist the skin in rebuilding collagen.

Eat the foods that nourish your skin, including essential fatty acids (EFAs) and plenty of vegetables and fruits daily. Avoid all junk food, alcoholic beverages, caffeine, and sodas. Even if you start eating well for the first time in your 50s, your face and skin will benefit.

Your skin could lack vitality. Now is the time to have fun with activities that revitalize your skin. Get outside more often while using plenty of sunscreen. You can also wear a sun hat and clothing with a high SPF rating. Enjoy vigorous activities, such as jogging, hiking, or biking. Increase your muscle mass and build core strength with exercise systems such as Pilates, yoga, and weight lifting. Increase bone mass with weight-bearing exercises, such as jogging, hiking, or walking. Regular massage and lymph drainage will help perk up your skin.

Now is a good time to consider a surgical facelift. This proves to be a good investment because the results can last up to 10 years. You'll look refreshed and relaxed. Be sure to shop carefully for a board-certified surgeon and understand the risks completely before you have surgery. You'll learn more about plastic surgery and choosing a plastic surgeon in Chapter 30.

Sixties and Beyond

Yes, you can have great-looking skin in your 60s, 70s, 80s, and beyond. For women, menopause has passed. Your skin is thinner, with heavier wrinkling. Lifestyle and genetic diseases and disorders, such as diabetes, high blood pressure, high cholesterol, and heart disease can affect the radiance of your skin.

This is when lifestyle makes the biggest difference in the quality of your skin. If you are eating low-glycemic foods, maintaining a healthy weight, and exercising regularly, your skin will radiate vitality and exude health. Plus, you'll be improving any health conditions you have.

Stay active and keep your attitude bright and cheerful. Develop new interests and pursue new hobbies and adventures. Yes, these have a highly positive effect on your overall well-being, and that shows up in the quality of your skin.

Keeping your skin dewy and moist is a challenge. You'll have more skin growths, as in skin tags, flesh moles, and perhaps skin cancer. Be sure to have your skin checked regularly by your health practitioner for growths and have them removed professionally. Your skin is bumpier and rougher, so keep cleansing, toning, and moisturizing twice a day. Exfoliate often to increase cell turnover rate.

Men's skin will show sun damage in these years. Wrinkling and expression lines are evident. Be sure to manage hair overgrowth on eyebrows, nose, and ears.

Great skin in your 60s and beyond is moisturized and vibrant. The skin may have some darker pigmentation, but for the most part it has an even tone. If you've used sun protection faithfully all of your life, you have less sun damage and your skin has remained smooth. You have crow's feet and expression lines, but no cross-hatch lines.

The Least You Need to Know

 ◆ Your skin changes with each decade of life.

 ◆ Every age of your skin poses challenges to attaining and maintaining better skin.

 ◆ Make it a habit to cleanse, tone, and moisturize daily and exfoliate regularly.

 ◆ At all ages, use sunscreen or sunblock to prevent sun damage and skin cancer.

Part 2

Basic Skin Care Routines

Your skin needs your loving care at least twice a day, morning and evening. It requires the same habitual maintenance that other parts of your body need, like your teeth, which need brushing twice a day, and your stomach, which needs feeding at least three times a day. To begin, you need to identify your genetic skin type: normal, oily, sensitive, oil-dry, or acne. Then you can set up a twice-daily skin care ritual.

Then you need to understand that the skin of your eyes, neck, and lips responds well to slightly different treatments than the rest of your face. Learn how to plump up lips, soothe lines and bags around your eyes, and keep your neck finely tuned and toned.

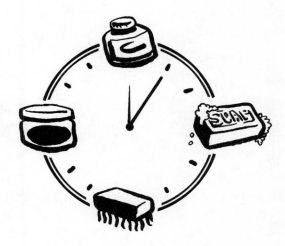

Uncover the Skin You're In

In This Chapter

- ◆ Discovering your genetic skin type
- ◆ About the five skin types
- ◆ Working with the skin type you inherited

Perhaps you've sighed at times as you thought, "Having great skin would be so simple if only I'd been born with it." Perhaps you've noticed that some people with terrific skin seem to do everything wrong. They live hard, miss out on sleep, eat junk food, and treat their skins with little, if any, care. For these lucky folks, burning the candle at both ends never shows up on their skins, whereas others do everything right and still struggle to maintain nice skin.

Blame it on genetics. Each of us was born with a specific type of skin and nothing can change that. It's like eye color. If a person is born with blue eyes, nothing can make them permanently brown. And vice versa.

Don't worry. In this chapter you'll find a questionnaire for determining your genetic skin type—the skin you were born with. Armed with that knowledge, you can start treatments and daily routines that will make your skin glow.

About the Genetic Skin Type Survey

Your first step to better skin begins with taking the Genetic Skin Type Survey. It will help you understand the intrinsic factors that shape the way your skin looks and behaves. This is the starting point for designing a daily skin care ritual that works best for you. Without this knowledge, your skin care regimen will most likely end up "hit and miss" and based more on luck and guesswork than on science and biology.

At different times in your life, your skin may need to be treated for skin conditions that are caused by extrinsic factors. These include sun damage, congestion and break-outs, or dark pigmentation. These treatments would be in addition to and in harmony with your basic skin care rituals for your genetic skin type. You'll learn all about these skin conditions and how to treat them in Part 4 of this book.

Body of Knowledge

You can blame genetics for the quality of your skin—but the blame only goes so far. No matter what type of skin you inherited, you can still have great and enviable skin. How? By using skin care and treatments based on leading-edge scientific knowledge and by making lifestyle changes in such areas as eating, exercise, environment, and supplements.

The survey covers basic skin types used by leading-edge skin care specialists. It's different from the questionnaires you may have filled out at the department store cosmetic counters. While cosmetic counter classifications may work well when purchasing skin care products, they aren't as helpful for understanding how your skin functions.

At the end of the Genetic Skin Type Survey, you'll get your results. You might be pleased, or you might be concerned. Don't worry needlessly. We explain each type, giving you both the benefits and challenges. Then, throughout the book, we'll tell you how your skin type works with the different treatments and procedures.

Genetic Skin Type Survey

As you take the skin type survey, answer each question based on how your skin has behaved throughout your life—from childhood, through adolescence, and on to adulthood. This will give you the most accurate typing. Your overall life experience with your skin and complexion is more important than the current snapshot of your skin condition, even if you are currently experiencing a difficult skin condition, such as premature aging or dehydration. We'll discuss difficult skin conditions and their solutions later in the book.

Genetic skin typing works for men and women. It works for peoples of all colors, national heritage, and age. It will work for you, too. To determine your biological and genetic skin type, answer the questions that follow with either a yes or a no. Remember, base your answers on how your facial skin has been over your lifetime— right now we're only concerned with your genetics.

1. Is your day-to-day skin supple and resilient? Supple and resilient skin is plump and springs back when touched, like a foam rubber ball does. You seldom get bags under your eyes or sagging skin. N

2. Does your skin have good elasticity? Here's a quick test for elasticity. Pinch the skin on the top of your hand for about 5 seconds. Release and notice how quickly your skin regains its normal shape. If it takes longer than about 3 seconds, your skin lacks elasticity. Y

3. Is the appearance of your skin translucent and radiant? Translucent and radiant skin seems to glow with light from within. N

4. Is it true that very few things disturb your skin's current state? This means that your skin in basically not affected by environmental pollution, smoking (not that we recommend smoking in any way), lack of sleep, caffeine, or junk food. N

5. Do you experience breakthrough oily shine within four hours of washing your face? N

6. Do your pores appear large? N

7. Is your skin thick and coarsely textured? N

8. Have you avoided premature aging? In other words, does your skin appear to be younger than your chronological age? N

9. Does your skin burn easily? Y

10. Do you blush easily when nervous? If you don't know the answer on this one, the answer's no. If you do blush easily when nervous, you would know by now. Y

11. Does your skin have a tendency to redness when exposed to wind or when washed with soap and water? Y

12. Do you have sinus problems and/or allergies? This indicates an inflammation response. N

13. Does your skin have a fine texture with relatively small- to medium-sized pores but is rough to the touch? If your skin feels like fine sandpaper at times, answer yes to this question. Y

14. Does your skin have both dry and oily patches? If you have normal T-zone oiliness and dryness on you cheeks, answer no to this question. But if you have unusually placed patches of either dry or oily skin, then answer yes. N

The T-zone.

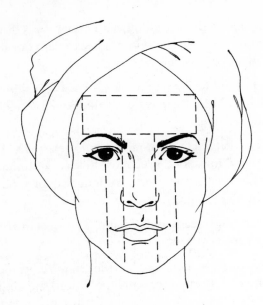

15. Is your skin dull or grayish?

16. Do fine lines appear randomly over your skin surface, as in crisscrossed or cross-hatched fine lines that aren't expression lines?

17. Do you have visible whiteheads and blackheads?

18. Does your skin have an uneven texture with raised bumps?

19. Does your skin tend to be active with pustules and cysts?

20. Is your skin often painful?

Body of Knowledge

You can understand your skin type by observing the skin of your parents, brothers and sisters, and blood relatives. Chances are that your skin is the same genetic type as one of them. If no one in your family has acne-type skin, chances are good that you won't either. The same is true for normal-type skin.

Here's how to score the survey. Count up all your yes answers. If your yes answers add up to:

1–4	You have normal skin.
5–8	You have oily skin.
9–12	You have sensitive skin.
13–16	You have oil-dry skin.
16+	You have acne-type skin.

Now it's time to learn more about the characteristics of your skin type.

Knowledge Is Power

As you read through this section, it's important to remember that skin knowledge is skin power. You may not like the type of skin you were born with. We sympathize. But look on the bright side. Any skin type *can* look radiant and beautiful. It's how you treat your skin that counts.

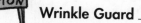

Wrinkle Guard

Don't be too concerned about what your skin type turned out to be. Instead, change your skin care methods and techniques to make your skin healthy and radiant.

Normal Skin

Lucky you. Most likely others envy your healthy, dewy, and moist skin. Although you may have occasional flare-ups, most of the time your skin stays balanced—meaning that it has the right amount of moisture to feel good and look great. It's healthily plump and tends not to wrinkle much, if at all. Your skin has a smooth texture and small- to medium-sized pores.

Your skin doesn't require lots of special treatments. Because it doesn't react dramatically, if at all, to environmental conditions, such as allergens, you can use a wide variety of skin care products without reacting negatively to them.

Your skin is considered to be the ideal. Persons with the other types aspire to have skin that looks as calm and clear as yours.

Skin-spiration

Cathy is 60 years old. Her daily skin ritual has stayed the same her entire adult life. She washes with soap and water, then applies an inexpensive drugstore moisturizer. Her skin is still dewy, moist, and radiant with no lines, wrinkles, or sagging. If she ever wants a more polished look, she dabs on a bit of pressed drugstore-brand powder. Cathy was born with normal-type skin.

Oily Skin

Oily skin has great advantages. Your skin is thick, and, as a result, it doesn't wrinkle much with age. Even if it thins as you age, you'll still appear to have a plumper skin than others your age. Oily skin seldom if ever feels dry and parched. Instead, it develops shiny patches a few hours after washing. You can keep the shine down with many of the great products now available such as blotting papers and oil-absorbing powders and foundations.

Oily skin often appears shiny with open pores. You may experience patches of break-outs on the chin or forehead. Your first challenge is to appreciate the oiliness to your best because it ultimately keeps your skin young and supple as you get older. Your second challenge is to control the oil with proper cleansing, toning, and moisturizing. You'll learn the specifics in the next chapter.

Sensitive Skin

Sensitive skin is thin skin. With aging, it develops fine-line wrinkles. You may have red capillaries around the cheek area with "hot" spots of red on the cheeks. Redness can occur from being outdoors in cold weather and from eating spicy foods. Oil glands can become inflamed, even though sensitive skin is typically not oily. Sensitive skin is more prone to rosacea than other skin types (see Chapter 13 for more information on rosacea).

Your challenge is to adopt lifestyle activities that keep your skin soothed and balanced. Plus, your key to better skin is to use skin care products and treatments that keep your skin balanced without irritation.

Oil-Dry Skin

Your skin is a challenge to you. You have visible dryness and flaking, with rough and patchy areas. Some areas may be tight and pulling. Your skin tone is uneven and your overall complexion appearance is dull. Your skin doesn't produce as much oil as other skin types, thus the designation oil-dry means your skin is dry due to lack of oil production. A clinical term for oil-dry skin is allapoid.

Oil-dry skin is a genetic condition and not due to environmental stresses or a dry climate. But certainly, environmental factors can make any type of skin appear dry due to dehydration. You can learn how to treat this skin condition in Chapter 14.

Don't despair. Your challenge is to make lifestyle changes and use regular skin care to calm and soothe your skin. By using skin lighteners you can reduce dark pigmentation, and light-reflecting foundations can even out both dark pigmentation and any redness. Your skin can appear dewy and the pigment evenly toned.

Oily/Acne-Prone Skin

Don't let the name of this category upset you. Many people with acne skin already have quite gorgeous complexions. And, if you don't now, you certainly can soon.

Acne-type skin doesn't mean you actually have acne or have ever had it in the past. It means your skin is genetically more prone than other types to disruptions such as blackheads, whiteheads, and pimples.

Acne-type skin easily becomes inflamed from using some skin care products and environmental stresses. Your skin seems inexplicably sensitive and vulnerable at times.

You need to exfoliate frequently, as acne-type skin doesn't exfoliate well by itself. If you don't exfoliate regularly, the skin becomes *keratinized*, and will require a more "heavy duty" physical exfoliant to regain its radiance. But be sure not to over-exfoliate because this can create more breakouts.

Clarifying Words

Skin becomes **keratinized** when dead skin cells build up and cover the newer skin underneath, leading to blemishes and dull skin. To remedy, use a physical exfoliant, such as cleansing grains. Use gently. (Details are explained in Chapter 5.)

There are six levels of severity for acne-type skin:

- Level One: Noninflamed. At the moment, the skin is calm and soothed with no breakouts, blackheads, or whiteheads. This skin can appear to be normal skin when cared for correctly.

- Level Two: Oily with blackheads and whiteheads. Your skin shines rather than glows.

- Level Three: Papules. Skin has small bumps, or pimples that are slightly elevated above the skin surface.

- Level Four: Pustules. Bumps larger than papules that contain pus.

- Level Five: Cystic. Cysts occurring beneath the skin surface are larger than a pustule and can become inflamed, leading to scarring.

Skin-spiration

Many people, just like you, are mastering acne-type skin and maintaining good-looking skin at level one. You can do this, too by using new skin care technologies and lifestyle modifications.

- Level Six: Active. All of the above happening at once. Can be active on both face and body.

For a person with acne-type skin, the challenge is to attain Level One status and maintain it. With proper care and treatment, and with proper lifestyle activities, you can do it.

Making the Most of Your Type

So no matter what your skin type is, get excited! By using the tools, techniques, and recommendations in this book, you'll start improving the quality of your skin today, and you'll see results virtually immediately—within days or weeks.

Soon, your skin could have such radiance and glow that others will ask you for your secrets.

The Least You Need to Know

- ◆ Genetics determines your skin type.

- ◆ Scientifically, your skin is classified as one of five skin types.

- ◆ Individuals of all skin types can have better skin by making the proper lifestyle changes and using the correct skin care.

- ◆ Cosmetics-counter skin classifications work for beauty products but may not be useful in understanding and caring for your skin.

Chapter 4

Wash, Tone, Moisturize ...
Wash, Tone, Moisturize

In This Chapter

- ◆ The benefits of daily skin maintenance
- ◆ Understanding cleansers, toners, and moisturizers
- ◆ Using sunscreen daily
- ◆ Tailoring a daily routine for your skin type

Think of an activity that you perform at least twice a day without fail. Perhaps you're thinking about brushing your teeth. But what about even more basic activities, such as eating? Chances are good that you seldom, if ever, forget to eat.

You need to make washing your face an activity as routine as eating. The good news is that, unlike eating, you only need to wash your face twice a day. With that minimal amount of effort, you'll be on the right path to healthy skin.

In this chapter, you'll learn why washing—plus toning and moisturizing—is so essential. Most importantly, you'll learn how to wash, tone, and moisturize for your skin type. Once you've established the proper routine of morning and evening skin care, you'll see results you can appreciate.

Take Two a Day

Establishing a basic daily skin care routine is the best thing you can do for your skin. Without twice-daily washing, toning, and moisturizing, other external treatments could be a total waste of time and money.

Notice that we say external treatments. Internal treatments include what you eat, how you exercise, and any vitamin and minerals supplements you take. These activities help create better skin from the inside out, and you'll learn more abut them in later chapters. But without a consistent regimen of external treatment these aids may not be effective.

External treatments include a wide range of skin products and salon or home treatments, and different products may be applied at different intervals. For washing, toning, and moisturizing, twice a day is ideal.

Wash Your Troubles Away

Overall, washing simply makes sense. Here's why. Washing your face and body in the morning removes the waste products released through your skin pores as you sleep. These can include external and internal toxins, sweat, and sebum. By simply washing your face, you help the body detoxify and thus purify both your body and your skin. This is essential for better skin.

In the evening, sometime before going to bed, wash your face again to remove the day's buildup of dust, environmental pollution, skin secretions, and sweat. Washing also removes foundation and other makeup residues.

> **CAUTION**
>
> **Wrinkle Guard**
>
> Make sure you don't use the same bar soap on your skin that you use on your body. Instead, use bar soaps specifically formulated to be used on your face. Many skin care lines offer bar soaps that work well to cleanse your face while keeping the pH of your skin balanced.

Washing prepares your skin for the application of moisturizers and/or sunscreens. It doesn't make sense to put fresh skin care products on dirty skin. Doing so merely traps dirt and dead skin cells and leads to clogged pores.

Plus, washing your face feels good. The water is refreshing and slightly stimulating. And we're all for feeling good.

You can wash you face with bar soaps, gel cleaners, or lotions, but make sure you use a skin-washing product that is specifically designed for facial skin. Otherwise, you may not like the results. Regular bar soaps can leave facial skin feeling tight and dry.

They can even overclean your skin and make it more susceptible to unwanted skin troubles because you strip away the acid mantle making it more difficult for your moisturizer to a good job. So wash twice a day and wash gently.

Most face cleansers today are pH balanced to assist your skin in maintaining the ideal acid/alkaline pH balance of 4.5 to 5. Keeping your skin slightly acidic protects it from external pollutants and chemicals. The acid mantle on your skin is your skin's first line of defense and keeps it moist and healthy. Using a cleanser too strong or too alkaline for your skin type or scrubbing too energetically can make your skin susceptible to annoying and potentially dangerous skin conditions.

One of the functions of sebum and sweat is to keep the skin's pH in balance. So keep on sweating, or as guys think girls say, keep on glowing!

Men, you may be getting by—or *think* you're getting by—washing your face using deodorant bar soap. However, you'll probably be surprised at how much better your skin looks and feels if you use a facial soap, gel, or lotion. You'll be happier with the end result if you go ahead and use a skin care product, and it doesn't really matter if it's designed for men or women—as long as you get the results you want.

Skin-spiration

The only way to find a skin care product that works best for you is trial and error. You can certainly gather suggestions from friends and experts, but you can only know for sure by testing the products on your skin. Whenever you can, ask for samples to try at home. Most good skin care lines—from those found in department stores to those available at drugstores, discount stores, and grocery stores—will gladly accept returns on products that don't work for you or give you bad results.

Virtually all of the skin cleansers on the market work quite well, depending on your skin type. Don't expect expensive products to be more effective than those bought at the drugstore. What's most important is to find the products that work best for you, your skin, and your lifestyle.

You can tell if a skin care line works well for you if you like the way your skin looks. Your skin should be clear, smooth, with enough moisture but not so much that your skin

Wrinkle Guard

Select skin cleansers, toners, and moisturizers from the same skin care line. They're designed to be used together and give you consistent results. If you mix and match brands, you might get lucky. However, it's more likely that you won't get the results you're paying for.

appears oily. If skin care products make your skin itch or burn or make it red or inflamed, select another brand.

Whichever products you choose, be sure to cleanse as directed. Otherwise, you simply can't expect great results. In Part 3, we'll give you some guidelines for selecting skin care products.

Tone, Tone, Tone Your Skin

Next up is toning. Sometimes it's tempting to think that you can skip this step, and you could, but it will be that much harder to achieve the results you're looking for.

In the past, the purpose of toning was simply to restore and balance the skin's pH. Today, toners are often humectants as well. Humectants work to bind moisture to the skin and make moisturizers work better. Many toners on the market today also include added nutrients, such as vitamins and minerals, that may give your skin further protection.

Clarifying Words

To **spritz** means to spray the toner on your face. Hold the atomizer or spray bottle about 12 to 14 inches from your face, close your eyes, and spritz your face two or three times. Feels refreshing and cooling.

You can use several different application methods for toner. You can *spritz* it on, splash it on, or apply it with a clean pure-cotton pad. Spritzing uses less product, so you may want to transfer your toner to an atomizer. And if some of the toner gets into your hair, don't worry, it's most likely good for it.

If you prefer using a strong cleanser that can destroy the acid mantle of your skin, then be sure to follow up with an acidic toner and apply with a cotton ball for complete coverage. It's thought that once the acid mantle is stripped, it will take your skin up to 36 hours to regain its correct pH from within the skin.

Moisturizer Makes a Difference

The final step in your twice-daily routine is to moisturize your skin. First of all, let's discuss what you can reasonably expect from a moisturizer, and what you can't. If we clear up some common misconceptions now, you'll have a more realistic idea of what a moisturizer can do for you, and you'll be happier with the results.

Many people think that if only they had the perfect moisturizer, they'd also have great skin. But skin doesn't work that way. A good moisturizer simply helps keep your skin moist, dewy, and protected throughout the day. It gives the skin *slip*, and allows the surface of your skin to feel hydrated and not tight or dry.

A moisturizer is wrong for you if the ingredients aren't harmonious with your body. If it gives you a rash, irritation, or redness, stop using the product immediately and switch to a moisturizer with different ingredients. We've included a list of ingredients that are most likely to trigger reactions in Chapter 22.

Clarifying Words

Slip is the sensation that the skin is smooth and ever so slightly slippery. Slip lets you apply foundation easily, allowing it to glide on smoothly and evenly. You have a healthy amount of slip when you touch your skin and your hand easily glides over the surface without catching on rough or dry patches.

Lightweight lotions usually contain humectants such as hyaluronic acid, glycerin, urea, or sorbitol that work by attracting water molecules to the skin. Heavier moisturizers contain ingredients such as petrolatum, mineral oil, shea butter, and cetyl alcohol that soften the skin and form a protective layer.

Many moisturizers also contain nutrients called cosmeceuticals, such as vitamins, minerals, and antioxidants. If your skin responds well to these ingredients, and doesn't show signs of negative reactions, then by all means use these product formulations.

If you live in a dry environment, such as the desert or the Rocky Mountain West, you may need a heavier moisturizer. The same goes for colder regions of the world such as Alaska and the northern United States in winter. But in areas of the country that have average to high humidity, a light moisturizer should suffice.

If you can't find a moisturizer that works for you, it's possible that none of them will be adequate until you make lifestyle changes that encourage moisture from the inside. Look at your lifestyle and determine what changes you need to make in order to improve and revitalize your skin. Part 5 of this book tells you how to create skin wellness through lifestyle choices.

Skin-spiration

Your skin has more moisture when you use a moisturizer designed for your skin type. But totally correcting dry skin isn't the job of a moisturizer. It's your job. You create skin moisture through your lifestyle—by eating well; by avoiding habits that harm your skin, such as smoking, drinking alcoholic beverages, and ingesting too much caffeine; and by proper exercise. When you do your part, a moisturizer can easily do its job of retaining skin moisture and protecting your skin from the environment.

Daily Sunscreen

The finishing step for your skin care routine is to apply sunscreen. You have many choices for sunscreen, but the most important thing you can do to apply it in the morning and then reapply again later in the day and especially before you go out into the sun for longer than 15 minutes.

Use a sunscreen with an SPF of 15 or higher. You can use a moisturizer with sunscreen, a foundation with sunscreen, or you can smooth on a sunscreen over your moisturizer.

The two kinds of sunscreens available are either chemical sunscreens or barrier sunscreens. A chemical sunscreen is absorbed by skin over two or three hours and needs to be reapplied before noon, and then again in the late afternoon. Chemical sunscreens allow the sun to reach the surface of the skin while using chemicals to prevent penetration and avoid sun damage.

A barrier sunscreen is also known as a sun block and contains either zinc oxide or titanium dioxide or both. Sun blocks sit on the surface of the skin and prevent the sun's rays from ever reaching the skin. Sun blocks last longer than chemical sunscreens because they aren't absorbed into the skin. You may only need to reapply once a day.

Skin-spiration

You can now purchase skin-enhancing lightweight powders that contain a SPF 20 sun block. These mineral makeups double as foundations or bronzers. The powder particles of zinc oxide and titanium dioxide are so small that they're only a fraction of the diameter of a human hair. You can reapply easily and quickly during the day simply by brushing on the sunscreen rather than needing to use messy creams and having to then repair your foundation and blush.

If you're concerned about the ultimate safety of applying chemicals to your skin, we recommend that you use a barrier sunscreen rather than a chemical sunscreen.

Be sure to apply an ample amount of sunscreen to your face and cover all areas, including your neck. Don't skimp on the sunscreen. You need protection all day long, not just when you are out in the sun. Seventy-eight percent of sun exposure comes from incidental light such as when you are driving a car, walking into the grocery store or office, or outside watering your plants.

Here are some suggestions for using sunscreen:

♦ Apply 20 minutes before going out in the sun and again after 20 minutes of sun exposure.

♦ Reapply every two hours, after swimming, after sweating, and after toweling off.

♦ Waterproof sunscreens last for 80 minutes in water and need to be reapplied after 80 minutes in the water. Water-resistant sunscreens last for 40 minutes. Reapply after 40 minutes.

♦ Give your nose a double dose of sunscreen. That's where most people develop sun-related skin cancers.

♦ Never use a sunscreen past its expiration date because it loses potency.

You can also use a foundation that contains sunscreen, but experts recommend that you also apply sunscreen before you apply foundation. In Chapter 16, you'll learn more about the research, the results, and how to guard against skin cancer, including using SPF protective clothing and nutritional supplements.

Daily Care for Your Skin Type

Each skin type needs slightly different products and procedures to assure healthy skin. To make sure that you're cleansing in a manner that's right for your skin, follow these recommendations, remembering that it's fine to make modifications based on your personal needs. Only you can really ever know what works best for your skin.

Normal Skin Daily Cleansing Ritual

Use any type of cleanser—bar, gel, or lotion. Even though you naturally have great skin, you still need to use a cleanser. Splashing your face with plain water isn't enough to nourish your skin and keep it clean. Follow the product directions for use. Wash morning and evening, applying cleanser to your face and neck.

Use a toner that contains a humectant and choose one that contains little to no alcohol. Use a light moisturizer in the morning and a richer, *nutrient-dense* moisturizer at night.

Clarifying Words

Nutrient dense refers to skin products that contain a high concentration of added vitamins, minerals, and antioxidants. These nourish the skin and provide added protection from free radicals.

Oily Skin Daily Cleansing Ritual

Your skin definitely needs cleansing twice a day. Use a stronger cleanser, such as a gel or facial bar soap. You can also use a daily cleanser that contains salicylic acid, which helps clear up blackheads and whiteheads. Be sure to lather gently over your entire face and neck, paying special attention to your oily areas, most likely in your T-zone.

Choose a toner that contains little to no alcohol. For oily skin, look for a hydrating spritz with ingredients including floral waters, aloe vera, or rose water. A toner with bioflavinoids is also good.

You definitely need an oil-free moisturizer when your skin is shiny with oil production perhaps through your thirties and even into your forties. Choose one that is *noncomedogenic* with humectants, and perhaps includes *silicone derivatives* such as cyclomethicone or dimethicone.

As you get older and your skin naturally gets drier, you can use a moisturizer with some oil and emollients.

Clarifying Words

Noncomedogenic indicates a type of skin care product that will not promote the formation of blackheads and whiteheads and won't cause breakouts. Some skin care products, such as lanolin, are comedogenic and can promote blackheads and breakouts. **Silicone derivatives** in moisturizers sit on the surface of the skin and lock in moisture without clogging pores and causing breakouts. They also give the skin a soft and smooth texture.

Sensitive Skin Daily Cleansing Ritual

Because your skin is sensitive, you may only want to cleanse once a day. It's important not to disturb your skin's pH balance, because that can make you susceptible to irritation. Use a lightweight lotion-type cleanser. Avoid heavy cold cream–type cleansers. If water disrupts your skin, find a cleanser that can be used without water. Select a cleanser with few and simple ingredients. Like all skin types, you may have to experiment to find the cleanser that works without disrupting your skin.

Tone by spritzing a light toner that also functions as a humectant. Avoid anything that could leave a greasy or oily film. A bioflavinoids spritz could work well. Choose a moisturizer with a silicone base or one that is formulated specifically for sensitive skin. Be careful, because some moisturizers may cause inflammation, and be sure to use one that locks in moisture.

Skin-spiration

Susan's skin was sensitive to everything. Her skin reacted to pollution in the air as well as to skin care products and perfumes. It flaked in odd places, itched in odd places, and could turn red and inflamed for seemingly no reason at all. Then she learned how to calm it down. She found products that soothed her skin. She improved her skin's resistance to upsets by supplementing her diet with plenty of vitamins, minerals, and good fats. Today, she has great-looking skin by carefully managing not only her skin, but also her lifestyle.

Oil-Dry Daily Cleansing Ritual

Cleanse twice a day with a lotion cleanser that doesn't disrupt your pH balance. If in doubt, check with the skin care line representative, or phone the company's 800 number, which should be listed on the package or on its website. Your skin requires the utmost gentleness, so it's best to avoid cleansing gels and bars. Definitely avoid soap.

For toner, choose a humectant spritz or apply with cotton pad. Use a heavier moisturizer both day and night. You can use a moisturizer designated as a night cream both day and night. Choose one that is nutrient dense. This is especially important at night, when your skin goes into "rest and repair" mode and can best utilize the nutrients.

Acne-Type Daily Skin Ritual

You need to clean twice a day and only twice a day. With this type of skin, avoid the temptation to cleanse more frequently, because this can overstimulate your skin and cause more breakouts. If you like, it's fine to blot your skin with blotting cloths when it appears oily during the day.

You need a stronger cleanser than the other skin types. The cleanser needs to be able to kill and eradicate the p. acne bacteria that cause breakouts. Look for products that contain salicylic acid or benzoyl peroxide. Other

Skin-spiration

Phyllis felt she looked older than her friends, and she was only 31. Her skin was oil-dry. Her skin needed plenty of rich emollient creams and gentle care so that she looked her age and not older. She applied cosmeceuticals, such as vitamins and other nutrients before bed. Her skin lost its surface dryness and began to radiate and glow.

ingredients that are effective against p. acne bacteria are sulfur and camphor. Your best choice is a gel-type cleanser or one made specifically for acne-type skin.

Choose a toner that contains salicylic acid along with a humectant. Apply with a spritz or a cotton pad.

Wrinkle Guard

If you have serious, active acne, by all means consult with a dermatologist. But if you simply have acne-type skin that's inactive or mild, you can usually manage it very well with good daily skin care plus a healthy lifestyle. Consider occasional visits for facials with a licensed skin care professional.

Make sure that your moisturizer is oil-free. That said, tea tree oil could be great for acne-type skin. When shopping, the rule of thumb is to select skin care products that are specifically formulated to work with acne-type skin. Your moisturizer needs to be noncomedogenic. Healing ingredients may include allantoin, cucumber, chamomile, amino acids, and trace minerals.

Less is more when using moisturizer for acne-type skin, so don't overdo it. You need enough so that your skin feels good and doesn't feel tight. But don't use a thick coating of moisturizer because your skin produces plenty of oil as it is.

The Least You Need to Know

◆ Your best daily skin care ritual includes cleansing, toning, and moisturizing.

◆ Persons of any skin type will enjoy healthier skin when using the daily ritual that matches their genetic skin type.

◆ Modern cleansers, toners, and moisturizers contain ingredients that improve skin health and moisture retention.

◆ Make daily skin care a high priority in your morning and nighttime hygiene—just like brushing your teeth.

Chapter 5

Exfoliation

In This Chapter

- ◆ How exfoliants benefit your skin
- ◆ Different types of exfoliants
- ◆ Choosing an exfoliant suited to your skin type
- ◆ Exfoliating your whole body

It seems like everyone—and every product—is doing it these days. Exfoliating, that is.

Exfoliation is a quick and effective health and beauty technique. In just a couple of days, your skin accumulates dead skin cells along with other natural skin waste products. As these waste products build up on the surface, your skin becomes dull and can appear sluggish and tired. Exfoliation is the application of products that remove this waste and restore your skin's natural beauty.

After exfoliation, your face feels smoother to the touch and has a more refined texture. Your skin will glow radiantly—provided you exfoliated correctly for your skin type.

In this chapter, we tell you all about the different kinds of exfoliants and which ones will work best with your genetic skin type. The afterglow will boost your confidence and make your skin look great.

The Ancient Miracle Product

Natural exfoliants have been with us for many centuries. Ages-old skin care techniques included clay masks and milk baths. You've heard of Cleopatra? It's recorded that she and other ancient Egyptians used natural exfoliants. In fact, it's likely that in-the-know cavewomen benefited from caches of mineral clay near riverbeds or lakes.

A couple minutes' rest with a mudpack on her face felt good, even if she didn't have the use of a mirror to admire her results.

We love exfoliants because they make all of us look good. In today's world, you can purchase excellent exfoliants at your local grocery, drugstore, or discount outlet. Fancier versions are available at department stores, spas, salons, and health food stores. Yes, we still use clay masks, but rather than trekking down to the local riverbed, acquiring a good exfoliant is as easy as a quick trip to the store.

Skin-spiration

Men exfoliate part of their facial skin every time they shave. However, you should still use exfoliants on the parts of your face that you don't shave, and it's always a safe bet to exfoliate your whole face whether you've shaved or not.

Properly Using an Exfoliant

Let "gentle" be your guideline when exfoliating. Go soft and easy and you'll like the results. Use a heavy hand or use an exfoliant too frequently and you'll need time out to heal from overindulgence. For some skin types, it's tempting to overdo it, but avoid this at all costs. You could create yet another skin problem. That problem is called cortisol overload. The stress of overexfoliating causes an increase in your cortisol levels. Too much cortisol is bad for your health and can lead to serious disruptions—not just in your skin, but throughout your body. So take it easy. The point is to soothe your skin, not punish it.

You know you've gone too far with an exfoliant if your skin turns red. Your face might also peel or flake. Leave the skin peels—as in heavy-duty chemical peels—to a trained professional.

If you ever accidentally overdo exfoliation, apply aloe vera gel or a washcloth dipped in soothing chamomile tea to the damaged areas. Both of these remedies are soothing and reduce inflammation and redness. Plus, they cool the skin and make it feel better.

You can find aloe vera gel at the health food store, or simply snip a leaf from an aloe plant and apply the somewhat sticky gel directly to your face. History tells us that the army of Alexander the Great pulled along wagons filled with aloe plants as they conquered Mesopotamia. The fresh aloe gel was great for healing battle wounds.

Wait until your skin is healed before exfoliating again. To help you avoid exfoliation mistakes, we'll spend time later in this chapter on recommendations for each skin type.

When to Exfoliate

The best time to use an exfoliant is when it's convenient for you—either morning or evening. First, cleanse your face, then apply the exfoliant. Remove the exfoliant, then continue with your daily ritual—toning and applying moisturizer.

Some exfoliants are included in cleansing products and in moisturizers. These combination products may seem to make life easier and your skin care routine simpler, but daily exfoliation isn't necessary for any skin type.

If you want to use a combined product, such as a cleanser with either a chemical or physical exfoliant, only use it two or three times a week. On the off days, use a non-exfoliating product.

However, the safest way to cleanse and exfoliate is to use products specific to the task. Use a daily cleanser that does not contain exfoliants, and on days when you choose to exfoliate, use a product specifically designed for exfoliation.

In Search of the Perfect Exfoliant

So many choices, so little shopping time. What's a person to do? If you've been shopping for skin care products lately, you've undoubtedly noticed the huge selection of exfoliants available and have probably read some of the labels. Confused? In this section we cut to the quick and give you the information you need to make a wise purchase.

There are essentially four types of exfoliants, each with its own benefits. Here's what you need to know.

Chemical Exfoliants

Chemical exfoliants dissolve the natural buildup of dead skin cells, sebum, and sweat, or what we refer to as "intracellular cement." They react with this cement to dissolve it and the waste products are then rinsed away. As such, chemical exfoliants need to be used carefully and with caution. Too much can burn the skin.

Chemical exfoliants are either alpha hydroxy acids, commonly referred to as AHAs, or beta hydroxy acids, known as BHAs. Both kinds are frequently used in the same product.

The most commonly used chemical exfoliants are:

- Glycolic acid, an AHA, made from sugar.

- Phenol, used only by physicians and paramedical technicians in chemical peels.

- Salicylic acid, a BHA, made from aspirin. Salicylic acid is the only exfoliant that helps kill germs as it clears your skin.

- Lactic acid, made from milk.

> **Body of Knowledge**
>
> Both salicylic acid and aspirin are derived from the bark of the white willow tree. When searching for a product that contains salicylic acid, you might find the ingredient listed as white willow bark.

Apply a thin layer of a chemical exfoliant to a clean face and neck, avoiding the eye area. Simply apply and let sit for a couple of minutes. You don't need to rub the product into your skin, as the chemicals do all the work.

Enzymes as Exfoliants

The pulp of certain fruits contains enzymes that actually can digest the dead skin cell buildup on the skin. Enzymes are chemicals that help digest foods and other substances. Your stomach secretes enzymes to digest food. The fruit enzymes have been used for many thousands of years as beauty treatments to "digest" dead skin cells. Papaya and pineapple are often used for exfoliation. Papaya contains the enzyme papain and pineapple contains bromelain. Pumpkin is another great choice for enzyme exfoliants. These work on the surface of the skin, and are great for skin with little bumps.

You can purchase papaya or pineapple fresh from the grocery store, mash some up, and apply directly to clean facial or body skin. It smells great, but can be a bit messy. Leave the pulp-mask on for 10 to 20 minutes, then rinse off. If you face starts to feel hot, rinse it off immediately.

Enzyme exfoliants can usually be found at health food stores, and at some boutique skin care shops. You may have a more difficult time finding packaged exfoliants at a drugstore, grocery store, or discount store.

Apply enzyme exfoliant in a thin layer to cleansed skin and neck, avoiding the eye area. Don't rub it in, just let it sit on the skin. Keep on your skin for 10 to 20 minutes, or as directed. Rinse off with water, then tone and moisturize as you would normally.

Exfoliant Scrubs

Scrubs feel grainy. Exfoliating scrubs are made with grainy substances that act to massage away the dead skin cell matter. Scrubs made with organic matter contain grainy substances such as ground nutshells, clay, cornmeal, oatmeal, or rice powder. Man-made grainy materials include polyurethane or silicone beads.

Some forms of organic scrubs aren't very good for your skin. Ground-up nutshells can be too rough and abrasive. They create *microlacerations* on the skin, which wounds the skin and can cause inflammation from microlacerations. Microlacerations take time to heal and leave the skin red and inflamed, and unfortunately, wounded skin is susceptible to infection.

Conversely, polyurethane or silicone beads are smooth, and they roll in and out of the pores very gently. This is also true for organic scrubs such as finely ground cornmeal. We recommend them.

We include clay masks, oatmeal, and rice powder as scrub exfoliants because they function to remove dead skin cells. They're very gentle and are excellent for certain skin types, and we'll get to specifics in a moment.

Use a small amount of scrub and apply it to your neck and face. Using small circular movements, rub gently on all areas of your face except the eye area. Be sure to include the sides of your nose, chin, forehead, and jaw line. Rinse well to remove all traces of the beads. Then tone and moisturize.

The "rule of pressure" in using scrub exfoliants is this: Let the product do the work. Your hands are only there to deliver the scrub to your skin. Use virtually no pressure; just move the scrub around your face, avoiding your eye area. Exfoliate your lips as well as your neck and *décolleté*.

Clarifying Words

Microlacerations are miniscule or tiny tears or scrapes on the surface of the skin which can be caused by using physical exfoliants that are too harsh, such as ground-up nutshells, buff puffs, or loofahs, and especially when using physical exfoliants.
Décolleté is the area in women from the base of the neck to the top of the bosom. We include this area in the section on facial skin. The décolleté is revealed when wearing simple V-neck T-shirts, tailored blouses, and evening wear.

Direction to apply scrub exfoliants.

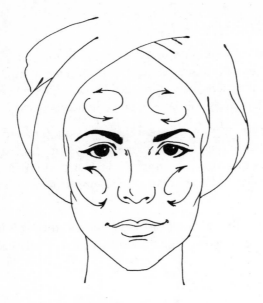

Mechanical Exfoliants

Although it's possible for you to use mechanical exfoliant machines at home, we don't recommend it. These machines remove dead skin cells, but they're tricky to use. It's easy to use too much pressure or to use for too long a period of time in one area. Both of these errors result in inflammation, microlacerations, redness, and even pain.

Examples of mechanical exfoliants are a hand-held microdermabrasion machine, rotating brush, or an ultrasound device. Using these machines correctly is difficult, and you could make a mistake that you'll regret. We don't recommend them for home use. These types of treatments are best left to professional skin care technicians.

Skin-spiration

As the population's use of exfoliants keeps growing, product manufacturers are creating more and more variations and combinations of the standard chemical, enzyme, and scrub exfoliants. Try to stay informed about new, innovative ways to exfoliate, keeping in mind the cautions mentioned in this chapter. Better informed is better skin!

Combination Exfoliants

You'll find exfoliant products in the stores that combine enzymes and scrubs, or chemicals and scrubs. They're fine to use if they don't irritate your skin and instead leave it looking clear and refined. Some are called gommages; others are lotions and creams.

Exfoliation for Your Skin Type

Each skin type has different exfoliation needs. As you begin to experiment with exfoliating, start with the following recommendations. Then you can determine if you need more or less exfoliation and make the adjustments that work for you personally.

These recommendations can't take into account your skin's own special needs. So go slowly and gently at first to learn what works best for you.

Normal Skin Exfoliation

Normal skin needs exfoliation about three times a week. You can use any type of exfoliant—chemical, enzyme, or scrub. You may prefer to use a combination.

Oily Skin Exfoliation

With oily skin, you may be tempted to exfoliate every day, thinking that the more exfoliation you perform, the easier it will be to control and reduce your oil secretion. In fact, just the opposite is true.

Daily exfoliation can overactivate your skin and make it even oilier. Instead, exfoliate a maximum of three times a week.

Any of the following products can work well for your skin:

- A clay mask. Apply the mask according to the package directions. Leave on your face about 10 to 20 minutes. Rinse.

- Salicylic acid. Look for products that contain salicylic acid and use as directed.

- Highly refined and finely ground cornmeal. You can purchase the cornmeal at the grocery or health food store. Mix a tablespoon of cornmeal with a bit of warm water. Apply gently to your skin and massage for a couple minutes. Rinse.

- Exfoliants with polyurethane or silicone beads. These are gentle and don't overstimulate your skin but do a terrific job of removing dead skin cells. Use according to the package directions.

◆ Enzymes. Use only a small amount and rinse thoroughly, being sure to get all of the product off your skin because they can continue to work for a long period of time.

Sensitive Skin Exfoliation

Yes, your sensitive skin needs exfoliation, but be careful. Your skin reacts unpredictably to skin care products, so you need a gentle exfoliant. Avoid chemical exfoliants as they can leave your skin red and inflamed. Instead, choose rice powders or old-fashioned oatmeal.

To use, moisten 1 or 2 tablespoons with a small amount of water. Put on skin, relax for 15 to 20 minutes, then rinse off.

The oatmeal softens dry, patchy areas and soothes inflamed skin. The rice powder gently removes dead skin cells without causing irritation. If you have sensitive skin, you should only exfoliate once a week.

Oil-Dry Skin Exfoliation

Your skin really needs exfoliation. In its natural state, your skin doesn't have enough sebum or oil. You want to stimulate oil production. You should still only exfoliate three times a week, but your skin can handle stronger exfoliants, such as glycolic acid AHAs or scrubs with polyurethane or silicone beads. Enzymes are also great for your skin type, especially for dry patches.

You may want to alternate use of glycolic acid, beads, and enzymes. First, cleanse your skin, then apply the exfoliant. Rinse off and follow up with toner and moisturizer.

Acne-Type Skin Exfoliation

If your skin is inflamed with active acne, use salicylic acid three times a week. Salicylic acid helps kill germs, and that's great for your skin. Clay masks and enzymes will also work well on your skin. You can also choose to alternate between salicylic acid, clay masks, and enzyme treatments. Always apply exfoliants to a clean face, and rinse well after using. Finish your routine with toner and moisturizer.

Exfoliation makes skin more active, so restrain yourself from exfoliating more than three times a week. You don't want active skin; you want soothed and calm skin. Avoid using scrubs, because they are too stimulating.

Notice how your skin feels and behaves after each exfoliation, then adjust the timing of your exfoliation and the type of product to get the best results.

The Rest of Your Body Wants Exfoliation, Too

Pamper yourself with all-over body exfoliation. The application stimulates your skin and feels great. Plus, it leaves your entire body—arms, legs, hands, and torso—soft and smooth.

Apply a body exfoliant in the shower or the bathtub. You can use the same chemicals, scrubs, and enzymes you use on your face, or you can choose to use products designed for body-use only, such as salt scrubs and sugar scrubs. They're luscious and feel quite indulgent, so give them a try. Exfoliate your body once or twice a week and you'll relish the results.

Another excellent technique for body skin exfoliation is dry brushing the body. You can use this method every day, because it offers light exfoliation along with healthy detoxification. Purchase a natural bristle brush and, each morning before your shower, gently dry brush your body. Start with your feet and work up your legs. Brush from your hands up your arms, and finish with your torso. It feels wonderful, gently removes dead skin cells, increases circulation, and stimulates lymph for detoxification. You'll learn more about the benefits of dry brushing in Chapter 22.

Skin-spiration

Planning a special beach vacation or romantic getaway? Be sure to pack along a luxurious body scrub. Your skin will love you for it and it can be wonderful fun to share with your spouse or partner.

The Least You Need to Know

◆ Exfoliants remove dead skin cells and other debris from your skin, leaving it smoother and softer.

◆ Correct use of exfoliants requires a gentle and loving touch.

◆ Choose an exfoliant that works best for your skin type.

◆ Use exfoliants all over your body for smooth and glowing skin.

Chapter **6**

Hair Removal for Men and Women

In This Chapter

- ◆ Exploring the many methods for removing hair
- ◆ Making shaving easier and more effective
- ◆ Products that can slow hair growth
- ◆ Hair-removal alternatives

Unwanted hair growth and its removal is one of the most groan-inducing topics in personal grooming. It can be tedious, time-consuming, and even painful. Perhaps you've wished it would just go away all by itself and that you'd never have to deal with it again. Instead, hair just keeps getting longer and more demanding every day.

Unless you're a man with a full beard, shaving is simply a fact of life. Women may not need to remove hair daily, but they're just as involved, if not more so, in hair removal as men.

People want and expect hair growth in some areas of the body, and remove it from others. Most of us want hair on our scalps. We expect men to be rugged and have facial hair that they shave. Many of us find a scruffy morning face to be masculine and sexy. And yet, we usually feel differently about a woman with hairy underarms or hairy legs.

In this chapter, you'll learn all about hair removal techniques—shaving, waxing, depilatories, and more. The fact is, you'll probably always need to spend time removing body and facial hair, but at least you can do it efficiently in a way that leaves your skin safe and healthy.

The Mystery of Hair

The mystery isn't that we have hair—it serves as protection for humankind, keeping us warm and protected from germs. And, although it varies across cultures, the mystery isn't that we desire to control where hair grows and where it doesn't on our bodies and faces.

No, the real mystery of hair is that no one really understands it from a biological or scientific point of view.

For example, no one can say for certain how it grows. Even if we think that all the hair follicles in a certain area of the body have been destroyed by electrolysis or laser hair removal, new hair can still grow. Sometimes the new hair sprouts from hair follicles that were previously dormant.

Hormone production plays a large role in where, how, and how much hair grows. Yet biologists cannot readily predict hormonal hair growth.

While we often wish for it, we've yet to discover a method of permanently removing hair, in large part because we don't completely understand it. Certain hair-removal treatments can aid in this, but can't totally eradicate hair growth. For example, waxing diminishes the quantity and thickness of hairs, but even when you've been waxing consistently for more than 20 years, hair still grows anew and needs to be removed.

Unless we come to a fuller scientific understanding of hair in the future, you'll just have to accept the fact that you'll regularly spend time removing it from your body. The good news is that there are various methods for doing so, and you should be able to find one that works best for you.

Shaving

The most common form of hair removal is shaving. Most men do it daily; women usually two or three times a week. Getting a good shave isn't easy, but by using the right equipment, the right preparation, and the right techniques, you can get a close, smooth shave every time.

Men shave their faces; women shave their underarms, legs, and sometimes their bikini line. But beyond the location, the differences end. The guidelines for shaving are the same for men and for women.

The Right Equipment

Shaving with the proper equipment is critical to a great shave and relatively simple. The first step is to purchase a razor that uses disposable razor blades. Avoid using plastic disposable razors. Though seemingly convenient, they simply can't deliver the results you're looking for.

You should able to keep a good razor for years, and should expect to change out the blades once a week. Always use a razor blade that has at least two blades. Three is even better. The multiple blades give you a closer and more even shave, and replacing dull blades is crucial. If you shave with a dull blade, you're far more likely to get ingrown hairs.

Make sure the handle of the razor is grooved or square—don't purchase a razor with a smooth, rounded handle. It'll be hard to grasp and hold steady while wet or coated with shaving cream or gel.

Plenty of Moist Heat

The secret to a great shave is to apply moist heat. Moist heat makes hair more pliable, and helps you avoid ingrown hairs. You'll also find moist heat makes it easier to shave.

Men can apply moist heat to their faces by wrapping a wet, hot towel around the face for several minutes until the skin softens, just like in the old-fashioned barbershop. Another method is to shave immediately after your morning shower. While you are washing, your face is steaming and softening. You can also shave in the shower. All you'll need is a shower mirror that won't fog up.

> **CAUTION**
>
> **Wrinkle Guard**
>
> Men, if you shave your head as well as your face, don't use the same razor for both. Keep one reserved exclusively for your scalp, and use a separate razor on your face. This prevents the possible spread of any scalp condition like dandruff to your face, and vice versa.

> **CAUTION**
>
> **Wrinkle Guard**
>
> Don't overdo the heat on your face. Avoid using a moist towel that is too hot—burning your face definitely won't help you get a great shave. Also, never use a blow-dryer to heat up your face or skin in preparation for shaving. The heat is drying and won't help you like moist heat will.

If you need to shave midday and don't want to take another shower, here's a simple trick that works well. Fill your sink with warm water. Bend over the basin and splash your face 20 to 30 times with the warm water, then proceed with your regular shaving routine.

Women can get the same benefits of moist heat by shaving towards the end of a shower, or during a bath.

Application of shaving cream or gel comes after moist heat. Shaving cream isn't a substitute for moist heat. It can't prepare your skin for shaving. It has an entirely different function.

Shaving Cream or Gel

The purpose of shaving cream or gel is to create a protective barrier between your skin and the razor blade. The cream or gel gives a slip to your skin that lets the blade glide evenly and gently.

Despite what they advertise, the magic of a great shave isn't in the shaving cream or gel, and almost any shaving product will work. Simply choose one that feels good and smells good and doesn't irritate your skin.

> **Skin-spiration**
>
> You might try a shaving cream or gel that contains silicone, as it gives a soft slip to your face and creates an excellent protective barrier between the blade and your skin. But, as with any product, if you notice any skin irritation you need to switch to a different product immediately.

The Right Technique

Using the right shaving technique lets you avoid scrapes and nicks. You're less likely to get ingrown hairs and you'll get a closer shave.

First of all, take a good look at the area you want to shave. If the area has long hair or a thick regrowth, trim the hair with scissors before shaving. This goes for men who may be shaving off a beard or moustache, as well as for women who are shaving their bikini area.

Next, look at the direction of hair growth. Ideally, all the hairs grow in the same direction, but it's rare that things work out that way. Hair often swirls, has cowlicks, and can even seem to grow back on itself. Don't panic. You may simply need to turn your razor to a different angle to shave these areas.

> **Skin-spiration**
>
> Men often tilt up their chins as they shave the neck area. This causes the hairs to retreat a bit into the skin and prevents a really close shave. Instead, hold your chin at normal level. That way, the neck hairs move out just a bit and you receive a closer shave.

For the closest shave, you should shave against the grain of your hair growth. For example, women would glide the razor up their legs, from the ankles to the knee. Men will typically draw the razor up the face, from the jaw line toward the cheek.

If you have a tendency to get ingrown hairs in the area you're shaving, then shave *with* the grain. If you want to be absolutely certain that you've had the closest shave possible, you can give yourself a "military" shave. First, shave in the direction of hair growth, then lather up again and shave against the grain.

Unless you have a really heavy or dark beard, shaving once a day should be adequate.

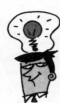

Skin-spiration

Women may be able to forego shaving their thighs if the hair growth is light-colored. The day-to-day friction of skirts, pants, and jeans actually removes hairs and diminishes hair regrowth.

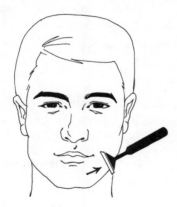

Shaving against the grain of hair growth.

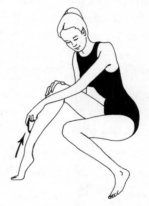

Woman shaving against the grain of hair growth.

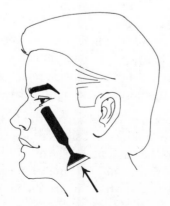

Correct way to shave neck.

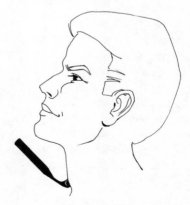

Incorrect way to shave neck.

To Splash or Not to Splash

After you've shaved, rinse the area well with water to remove any residue of shaving cream or gel. Rinse out your razor, or wash it.

At this point, you don't need to do anything more than towel dry your skin. Your skin doesn't require an aftershave for health or beauty reasons. However, if a splash after-shave feels good, then by all means use it.

Women can moisturize the shaved area with a light lotion that doesn't contain irritating ingredients.

Electric Shavers

Do you have light hair growth? Do you need a quick hair-removal touch-up? If so, an electric shaver could work well for you. But electric shavers aren't a good choice if you want to be impeccably groomed. Think of them as convenient. Using an electric shaver is quick, doesn't require water or heat, and the technique is simple. But you won't get as close a shave as you would with a razor.

If a man has a light beard, he can alternate using a razor with an electric shaver. He can give himself a great shave one day, and then use an electric shaver for touch-ups for the next day or two.

If you want to take a vacation from shaving on the weekends, as many men do, consider using an electric shaver for touch-ups.

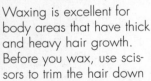

Skin-spiration

Waxing is excellent for body areas that have thick and heavy hair growth. Before you wax, use scissors to trim the hair down to a $1/4$ to $1/2$ inch in length. Then wax. As you continue to wax regularly for about a year or two, the hair will thin out and regrowth will slow down.

Waxing

Rip. Ouch. Sting. Why do we do this? Because it works. Waxing is here to stay. After all, what's a little bit of minor discomfort when you consider the rewards: being hairless for up to eight weeks at a time between waxings; not messing with razors and frequent maintenance; softer and lighter hair regrowth.

Waxing removes hair straight from the follicles. This damages the hair follicle and slows down regrowth. When regrowth occurs, the hair grows out thinner and finer. Over time—and by time we mean a year or two—you'll have fewer hairs in areas you wax.

Begin by waxing every two or three weeks, and then, as hair regrowth slows, you can wait longer in between waxings. After one to two years of repeated waxings, you may only need to wax once every eight weeks.

One disadvantage to waxing is that hair needs to be at least ¼-inch long in order to wax. You need to let yourself get a bit hairy before you can wax again.

You can wax any body area you choose—many women wax legs, underarms, and bikini area. Waxing also works well for facial hair on the upper lip and chin. Some women even wax their eyebrows. If you do this, make sure you absolutely know what you're doing. You don't want to be walking around with missing eyebrows for six to eight weeks!

Plenty of men wax their upper backs and other areas, such as the bikini line, but men seldom wax facial hair.

CAUTION Wrinkle Guard

Avoid waxing any part of the body where you apply Retin-A. Do not wax if you have been on an extended round of antibiotics or have used the prescription medication Accutane in the last six months. Check with your doctor or skin care specialist to determine how long you need to wait between the time of treatment and waxing. Stop exfoliating with AHAs or BHAs at least three days prior to waxing. Also, avoid waxing for six to eight weeks after a chemical peel and if you are using antibiotics. By taking these precautions, you can avoid irritating or damaging your skin.

You can wax your hair growth yourself by purchasing at-home waxing products at drugstores, grocery stores, and discount chains, or you can have it done at a skin care salon.

If you choose to wax at home, we strongly urge you to have it done at least once at a salon. You'll be better prepared for the experience, ready for that anticipatory moment when the wax is already on your skin and your only choice is to go ahead and rip it off. Rip. Ouch. Sting.

The three most popular product choices are as follows:

- Hard wax

- Soft wax

- Cold wax

Other waxing products are available at stores and on infomercials. You may need to try several before you find the product that works best for you.

Prep your skin before you wax. First, cleanse skin to remove oil and other residue from moisturizers and sunscreen. Dry your skin. Apply a protective barrier to the area. A simple and effective barrier is refined cornstarch. Use a very light dusting. The cornstarch slightly pushes each individual hair up and away from the skin, making it easier for you to see the hairs.

If you are using hard wax, be sure to read the package directions carefully before applying. Heat the wax until it becomes a liquid, but it still at a temperature that is comfortable to the touch, then apply the wax directly to your skin against the direction of hair growth. Wait until the wax cools and hardens, then remove by pulling away from skin in whichever direction seems easiest. The direction you pull off hard wax doesn't matter.

Apply soft wax, whether hot or cold, in the direction of hair growth. Put fabric strips over the wax. Grasp the strips firmly and quickly pull level against the hair growth.

You definitely will have an "afterglow" after waxing. Waxing removes the top layer of skin, meaning it's time to apply a cooling and healing lotion or gel to your skin. Not only will it feel good, you'll reduce the sting and avoid getting ingrown hairs. Good choices are products that contain tea tree oil or aloe gel.

For three days after waxing, avoid heat or overstimulation of the skin. That means no sun, no hot tubs, and no steam room. Also avoid exfoliating the area for three days.

Depilatories

Depilatories are lotions that contain strong chemicals such as calcium hydroxide and sodium thioglycolate. These chemicals dissolve hair growth above the surface of your skin. Use these products on your legs and underarms, but don't *ever* use them on your face.

The hair will grow back in a day or two, just as in shaving, so you'll need to use a depilatory two or three times a week.

In general, we don't recommend using depilatories. Repeatedly putting strong chemicals on your skin may not be great for the overall health of your skin or the rest of your body.

CAUTION Wrinkle Guard

Never use depilatories on your face. The chemicals are way too strong and can burn your skin, causing visible skin damage that can be very difficult, if not impossible, to correct.

Mechanical Hair Removal

You can now mechanically whir or tweeze away unwanted body hair. Mechanical devices, such as the Epilady or Silk-Epil by Braun, are fashioned like an electric shaver. However, unlike a shaver, which removes hair above the skin, mechanical devices grasp the hairs and pull them out at the roots. They do this quickly and, actually, quite efficiently.

These devices have gained something of a bad reputation because the process can be a little painful. However, it's not really any more uncomfortable than waxing, and, like waxing, it reduces and thins hair regrowth over time. But unlike waxing, hair removal with mechanical devices doesn't remove a layer of skin, nor does it involve potentially messy products, fabric strips, or clean up.

As with waxing, use a healing and cooling lotion or gel to soothe skin after using a mechanical device.

Zapping Away Unwanted Hair

Two different hair-removal techniques work by zapping hair at the roots, the idea being that the process destroys the hair follicle and prevents further hair growth. Alas, neither electrolysis nor laser hair removal are guaranteed as permanent solutions, but they can be effective in removing hair and inhibiting regrowth.

The effectiveness of both electrolysis and laser hair removal depends on how your body hair grows and how your skin reacts to this much stimulation. Although some people require only a couple sessions to see great results, others may need to have many sessions and will still have heavy hair regrowth. The results depend on the individual and are impossible to predict.

You are most likely to be successful with laser hair removal if you have light skin and dark hair. If you have light skin and light hair, ask for a treatment that combines radio-frequency waves with pulsed light. If you have darker skin and dark hair, laser hair removal is more likely to cause skin discoloration and dark pigmentation. Expect that it takes four to six sessions spaced four weeks apart to see an 80 percent reduction in hair regrowth. Per session you can expect to spend $1,000 for legs, $300 for the bikini area, and $2,000 for your upper lip.

Electrolysis can work well for people who aren't good candidates for laser hair removal, such as people with darker skin and dark hair or for people with light hair and light skin. But electrolysis can work for all hair and skin types provided that you don't scar. Be sure to have the technician do a patch test to determine if your skin is prone to scar from electrolysis. Electrolysis requires 15 to 30 visits for the upper lip. Expect to pay about $60 per 30 minute visit.

Before you sign up for electrolysis or laser hair removal, discuss the likelihood of your success with an expert at the clinic or salon. Ask for referrals of satisfied and unsatisfied clients and talk directly with them. Be sure to ask the person if they would do it all over again and if the results were worth the time and expense.

You can do electrolysis for yourself at home, but it's not easy. The home-use machines have less electrical current than those used at the salon. To destroy the follicle, you need to locate the follicle for each individual hair and zap it with the needle. It's difficult to be precise with hair on your legs and bikini area, and it's virtually impossible if you're self-administering to your back or underarms.

If you are still convinced that you want to try home electrolysis, you may want to have a professional session first to learn the ins and outs of this technique.

Laser hair removal can only be performed in a professional studio by a trained and licensed technician. This method can cause permanent skin discoloration (either lightening or darkening), swelling, inflammation, and infected hair follicles. If you have a tan or darker skin, beware, you could be at greater risk. Laser hair removal may permanently discolor your skin.

The biggest drawbacks to these techniques are that they're tedious, time-consuming, and, if done in a skin care studio, expensive. All factors considered, we don't think they work much better than waxing.

Other Hair-Removal Choices

Yes, there are even more choices for removing and managing unwanted hair. The following are four less common alternatives:

◆ Tweezing. This can be very effective for managing small areas of hair growth, such as eyebrows, the chin, and upper lips. Tweeze one or two hairs at a time. Use the best tweezers you can buy. Good tweezers make a big difference in accuracy and speed. Tweezerman makes the best and you should expect to pay between $5 and $25 for tweezers that last a lifetime.

◆ Stringing. This technique comes to us from the Middle East. It's inexpensive and all you need is a spool of sewing thread. Plus lots of know-how. By twisting the thread around several hairs at once and tugging quickly you pull the hairs out by the roots. This technique also reduces hair regrowth. People who master stringing swear by it. We doubt that anyone can easily learn this technique by reading a book, so you need to learn from an expert. To find a stringing expert, check your Yellow Pages under Hair Removal.

◆ Bleaching. While this isn't exactly a hair removal technique, bleaching makes it look as if you don't have the hair, so we included it here. Good for women's upper lip. Purchase hair-bleaching products at the drugstore, grocery store, or discount chains. It only takes about 10 minutes and lasts for a week or two.

◆ Hair-growth inhibitors. These over-the-counter products have come on the market in the past four or five years claiming that regular application can slow hair growth. Out on the street, the buzz is that they simply don't work. We question the metabolic and health wisdom of trying to stunt hair growth chemically.

◆ Vaniqa is a prescription drug that slows facial hair growth in women. Side effects include mild and temporary skin irritations such as redness, stinging, burning, tingling, or rash. But if heavy facial hair is a big concern for you, by all means, talk with your dermatologist, because you could get good results.

You may want to use these techniques on some areas of the body and not on others. Most people use a patchwork approach to hair removal or—some tweezing here, some shaving there, waxing in the summer, bleaching on the upper lip. Put together a patchwork that's best for your type of body hair and one that meets your lifestyle needs.

Ingrown Hairs

An ingrown hair is a hair that hasn't broken through the surface of the skin through the hair shaft opening. Instead, it continues to grow under the skin surface. When this happens, bacteria, pus, and dead skin cells get trapped along with the hair. The result is an inflamed bump.

Virtually all hair-removal methods can cause ingrown hairs, with the possible exception of depilatories. By using the techniques described previously for each method, you can reduce or eliminate ingrown hairs. But if your skin and hair are such that you easily get ingrown hairs, they may still occur.

> **CAUTION**
>
> **Wrinkle Guard**
>
> An ingrown hair can seem like a pimple, but instead, it's a hair that's just starting to grow back after hair removal. The hair gets trapped under the surface of the skin and continues to grow. This causes redness and traps the pore's natural excretions of sebum along with it. Picking is tempting but can make the situation worse.

Ingrown hair.

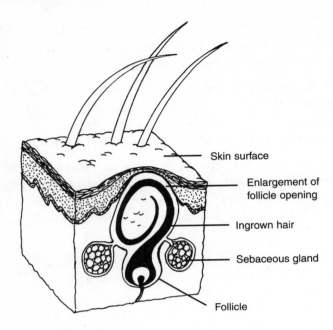

- Skin surface
- Enlargement of follicle opening
- Ingrown hair
- Sebaceous gland
- Follicle

First and foremost, refrain from picking at ingrown hairs. You could create bigger problems, such as infection and scarring. Instead, apply salicylic acid (BHA) to the ingrown hair with a Q-tip. An effective product for ingrown hairs is Tend Skin, which is available at salons and beauty supply shops. If you seem to get a lot of ingrown hairs, wait about three days after hair removal, then dip a cotton pad in a salicylic product and apply to the area.

At any time, you can use a plastic net or natural loofah to gently exfoliate the area. You can also dry brush the area daily before your bath or shower. You'll learn more about the technique and the health benefits of dry brushing in Chapter 22. These techniques help reduce the occurrence of ingrown hairs.

Skin-spiration

If you are prone to ingrown hairs after shaving, you may want to apply a salicylic acid lotion right after shaving. You can also apply a medicinal cream such as Neosporin right after you shave because it also can help prevent ingrown hairs.

The Least You Need to Know

- Hair removal isn't permanent, but it's sure here to stay.

- You can easily get a great shave by using the proper techniques and tools.

- Over time, waxing reduces the density and intensity of hair growth.

- Other hair-removal methods, such as stringing, bleaching, and tweezing can give you good results.

- Avoid and manage ingrown hairs with the application of salicylic acid and the use of a loofah or dry brushing.

Chapter 7

Special Care for Eyes, Lips, Neck, and Hands

In This Chapter

- ◆ Special care for special facial areas
- ◆ Protecting the delicate eye area
- ◆ Sustaining totally kissable lips
- ◆ Preserving a strong and supple neck
- ◆ Maintaining soft and lovely hands

Research and everyday observation tell us that not all facial skin is created equal. Some areas of your face require special care and attention. Similarly, the routine daily care of washing, toning, moisturizing, and periodic exfoliating is somewhat different for your eye area, lips, and neck.

These three areas have different textures and tend to age faster. Thankfully, caring for these areas doesn't require big changes to your basic routine, but a small amount of special daily and weekly treatment goes a long way toward perking up your skin's overall appearance.

In this chapter, you'll learn how to care for your eyes, lips, and neck to keep them looking great no matter what your age. We've also included information on how to care for your hands. Hands are exposed to the elements more than any other part of the body. They need loving attention to feel soft and to stay looking young and healthy.

The Windows to the Soul

Your eyes reflect your inner self to the world. Look deep into a person's eyes and you can see his or her natural radiance. At times, this radiance is mysterious, at other times, open and inviting. Eyes speak without words and can fill volumes with the single bat of an eyelash.

It's not only your eyeballs, but also the skin around your eyes that communicates. Ideally, that skin appears smooth, soft, and unlined, but it takes special routine maintenance to achieve these results.

Delicate Skin in Your Eye Area

The skin that's considered the eye area is in the hollow of the eye socket—the bone around the eyes. It extends from your eyebrows to the bones under the eyes, and from the bridge of your nose over to your temples, where smile lines develop if you smile a lot (and we hope you do).

The skin that covers the eye socket has very small pores. It's also thinner than the other skin on your face. The skin on the outer sides of eyes near your temples is more similar to the facial skin on your cheeks and forehead, but it's prone to early expression lines and the so-called and somewhat dreaded "crow's feet."

Before you worry too much about crow's feet, know that everyone gets them. Yes, a surgical eye tuck at the right time can reduce and soften their size, but you won't be able to escape crow's feet entirely. However, if you treat the skin around your eyes with loving care, you'll be able to weather the aging storm well.

Cream for the Eye Area

Using the same moisturizer on your eye area that you use for your face usually doesn't work very well. A face cream is too rich for this delicate area.

Using a rich cream can cause milia, which are small whiteheads, in the skin close to the eyes. Also, a rich face cream travels and migrates around the skin, meaning it can get into your eyes and cause irritation. The best way to get rid of milia if they haven't gotten hard is with a salicylic acid exfoliant. But usually by the time you can see milia, they're already hard. In that case, have them extracted by a profession skin care technician.

Wrinkle Guard _____

If you wear contact lenses, definitely avoid applying a rich cream to your eye area. It can travel into your eyes and cloud your contacts, thus impairing your vision. Rich cream is often impossible to get off contact lenses. When that happens, about all you can do is replace the dirty lens with a new one. Also, rich creams applied near the eyelashes can clog the tear ducts and prevent proper lubrication of your eyes.

Use a product that is specifically formulated as an eye cream. These products are designed to be light enough for the eye area, yet still deliver a high level of moisturization. They won't travel or migrate. The ideal cream firms and energizes as well as moisturizes. You only need to use a small amount of moisturizer—there's not a lot of surface to cover in the eye area and just a drop or two is plenty. Apply an eye moisturizer morning and evening as part of your daily routine maintenance.

Direction to apply eye cream.

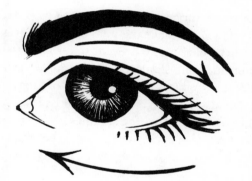

Apply a small amount of moisturizer in a light tapping motion around the eye. Start with the outer edge of the eye and tap the eye cream in toward the eye, being careful not to get the cream too close to your lashes. Eye cream migrates and moves, so some will spread up closer to your lashes. If some cream gets into the tear ducts along your lash line, it can block important eye excretions, causing dry eyes and, ultimately, boils. Tap eye cream on your upper eyelid, moving in toward the corner of your eyes.

Wrinkle Guard ____

Avoid using Retin-A in your eye socket area. You can use it outside the eye socket toward the temples, but avoid using it any closer to the eyes. Retin-A migrates and can irritate and cause damage to your eyes.

Eye Area Concerns

As much as we may not like it, the eye area is often a clear reflection of our lifestyle. A late night dancing into the wee hours shows up the next morning as under-eye bags or swollen eyelids.

Certainly, we all love cover-up or concealer for its temporary ability to mask the problem, but the underlying issues still exist. Here are some suggestions for your eye area concerns. They work equally well for men and women.

- Dark circles under the eyes. Yes, the tendency can be inherited, but there's plenty you can do about it. This area accumulates bodily waste products. To clear them out, get your lymph moving. Energize the area by dry brushing your body, perform a lymph-drainage facial, and use detoxification methods as detailed in Chapter 23. Yoga can work wonders to dissolve under-eye circles. It takes a couple of months to see results, but you may never need an under-eye concealer again.

- Baggy eyes. For temporary relief, use green tea bags soaked in water or slices of cold potato. Lie down and place the item over your eyes for about 10 minutes. Sleep with your head elevated to prevent water and wastes from pooling in eye area. During your morning skin care ritual, apply a firming product that puts a "seal" on the skin and reduces the appearance of saggy skin. Bags are sometimes hereditary and can also be the result of health issues, such as chronic allergies. Go to an allergist and get tested for allergies, especially to yeast, dairy, alcoholic beverages, and wheat. Cut back on caffeinated beverages, alcoholic beverages, diet sodas, and salt. See Part 5 for more information on making lifestyle changes to aid in the appearance of your skin.

- Fine lines. Use a hydrating moisturizer and you'll minimize their appearance. A firming product can really go a long way to diminish the appearance of fine lines. If the time comes that you feel it necessary, consider an eyelift.

- Crow's feet. Keep this area exfoliated and well moisturized. Use Retin-A, if desired. Keep smiling.

Use a concealer with a light-reflecting quality. It makes the eye area appear fresh and energized even after a late night. Avoid concealers in fancy colors, such as green, yellow, or pink. These are designed for photography and they're really hard to pull off in the full light of day. You'll probably just wind up looking like you smeared green or yellow goo under your eyes. Who needs that?

Fresh Lips

If the eyes are the window to the soul, lips are an indicator of youthfulness and sex appeal. Full, moist lips signal health and vitality. You can improve the lusciousness of your lips before you even apply lip pencil and lipstick.

As we age, lips get thinner, lose their plumpness, and fade in color. By using the suggestions in this section, you can revitalize your lips to make them appear more succulent, regardless of your age.

Exfoliate

Use a chemical exfoliant for the area of skin around your lips. You can do this at the same time you exfoliate your face. This is the area that develops small lines pointing toward the lips—often a sign of being a smoker. Smoking is never a good idea and is absolutely destructive to radiant skin. Those small lines also appear, though much more slowly, as we age. Lipstick can bleed into this area and make a person look ungroomed and a bit sloppy.

By exfoliating around your lips, you can smooth the area and reduce the appearance of lines, as well as help rebuild the underlying collagen.

Exfoliate your lips with a gentle scrub. Go easy. As you do this, your lips will receive stimulation from the increased blood flow. We think it tends to make the lips look fuller. Exfoliation removes dead skin cells, uncovering the redder color of healthy lips.

Wet Your Whistle

Your lips crave moisture. Lips have very tiny pores and hair follicles, although they're virtually invisible. Most of the moisture your lips receive comes directly from the products you apply. Licking your lips does moisten them for a while, but, ultimately, it can dry them out and leave your lips chapped.

Lipstick, lip gloss, or lip balm all keep your lips moist. Some contain natural humectants, such as honey, that are great for plumping up the lips. If you love the great outdoors, be sure to wear a waxy, ChapStick–type product

Wrinkle Guard

You use lipstick or a lip balm to protect your lips and make them look attractive. What's *not* attractive is repeatedly applying them in public. Don't reach for your lip protection the moment you feel the urge when you're in public. Apply it in private whenever possible.

with sunscreen when you're out in nature. On other days, find a lip protection product that doesn't dry out your lips. Choose a color or tint you love and apply as often as needed.

Your lips also need sunscreen, just as your skin does. Most of the lipstick-type products available today provide protection in the form of moisture and sunscreen, usually with an SPF of 15. Be sure to apply frequently, especially during sun exposure.

Go ahead and experiment to find a formulation that suits you.

An Inside Job

Lifestyle factors, especially your thoughts and attitudes, play an important role in the lusciousness of your lips. Thinking happy thoughts keeps your mouth relaxed and prevents wrinkling. Dwelling on unhappy situations and difficult relationships can actually lead to mouth wrinkles.

Releasing stress on a day-to-day basis can prevent the frowning and mouth tension that comes from feeling pressured. See Chapter 22 to learn more about how to master stress.

A Graceful Neck

No matter what shape your neck is in, you can make positive changes that will help to give you a lovelier neck. You can achieve tighter skin and reduce, if not totally eliminate, a double chin.

Ideally, your neck looks lean and strong. You can wear virtually any neckline and love the way your neck looks. You can enhance the suppleness of your neck with necklaces and earrings and feel comfortable. To achieve these results, your neck requires its own care in order to appear radiant and healthy.

> **Skin-spiration**
>
> Nothing makes a person look older than a double chin. You can get rid of a double chin with simple daily exercises that take less than 5 to 10 minutes. Plus, you'll look 20 pounds lighter. Do the Fountain of Youth exercises as described in Chapter 24 and you can bid adieu to a double chin in only three months.

The skin on your neck and décolleté is thin. When you care for your face, include both your neck and décolleté. Wash, tone, exfoliate, moisturize, and apply sunscreen.

Choose a toner that contains humectants (moisture-binding ingredients). You can use the same moisturizer that you use on your face, or you might try a moisturizer that's specifically formulated to firm the neck.

Be sure to use sunscreen on both neck and décolleté. It's easy to forget to apply sunscreen to your décolleté, but this area is especially vulnerable to the aging effects of the sun, so use sunscreen liberally.

Men who shave automatically take good care of their necks, because the act of shaving exfoliates the skin. Splash with toner if you like, but your shaving cream or gel already helps condition your skin. However, you do need to be sure and apply sunscreen to this area on a regular basis.

Silky Smooth Hands

Your hands go everywhere. They're on top of the steering wheel, getting a sunbath through the windshield. They're in water many times throughout the day. They wield a hammer, type on keyboards, lift snow shovels, and fold the laundry. Your hands seldom get to rest.

For most of us, the wear and tear shows. We get age spots related to sun exposure. Our nails break or split. Hang nails show up from time to time. The skin gets rough. All this in spite of the fact that we try to keep our hands lubricated and protected.

Hands are miracles of work and design, but they're miracles in need of some special TLC—tender loving care—from time to time.

Basic care for you hands should seem familiar by now:

◆ Exfoliate regularly. This makes hands baby soft and smooth. Use exfoliating products and dry brush daily. Learn more about dry brushing in Chapter 23. Exfoliation and dry brushing are great for your feet as well.

◆ Moisturize. Keep applying moisturizer throughout the day. Put jars or bottles of moisturizer at every sink, near the bathtub, in your car, and at your desk. You can use either a lotion or a cream, but search until you find one that works best for you and then use it regularly and liberally.

◆ Apply sunscreen. This helps eliminate the formation of age spots and reduces uneven pigmentation, so hands are evenly toned. Sunscreen also protects your skin. If you prefer, use a hand cream that contains sunscreen.

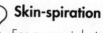

Skin-spiration

For a special nighttime softening treatment for your hands, apply a rich moisturizer, put on a pair of gloves, and go to sleep. In the morning, you'll have soft and supple hands. Plain petroleum jelly works well and is quite economical. This nighttime treatment is also great for feet. Slather with cream or petroleum jelly and then pull on cotton socks.

Your hands speak with you. They express you. Have them express your radiance and beauty with good daily care.

The Least You Need to Know

- Care for the delicate skin near your eyes with a light eye cream.

- Exfoliate and moisturize to keep your lips looking full and sensual.

- Treat your neck and décolleté at the same time that you care for your face.

- Give your hands continual daily protection with liberal use of both hand cream and sunscreen.

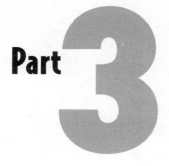

Part 3

At the Store: Cosmeceuticals and Skin Care Products

Walking into a store to purchase skin care products can be intimidating, whether you are shopping at a high-end department store or at the local discount chain. There are so many products, so many skin care lines, so many product claims. How does a person know where to start, let alone what to buy?

In this part of the book, you'll learn some insider secrets. You'll learn all about cosmeceuticals, and what you can reasonably expect from skin care products. You'll learn the difference between expensive and inexpensive products and that often price has more to do with packaging, brand name, and promotion than the actual value of the ingredients.

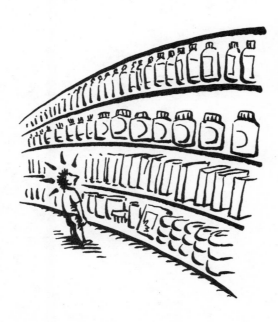

Chapter 8

What's in Your Skin Care Products?

In This Chapter

- Learning to read the product label
- The importance of cosmeceuticals
- What ingredients are doing (and not doing) for you
- The risks of going natural

So skin care products are supposed to be good for you, but what's in them? If you're reading the label of a skin care product, it can be difficult to tell. The ingredient list looks like it's written in Latin, but it might as well be Greek to most of us.

Today, the ingredients in over-the-counter skin care products are often a combination of cosmetics and cosmeceuticals. Cosmetics are less than skin deep. They don't actually change the skin, but they can add moisture and help make your skin look good. Cosmeceuticals truly change your skin for the better, but aren't as strong as prescription medications.

In this chapter, you'll learn not only how to read a product label, but also how to understand what you're reading. With knowledge comes power. This chapter puts you in control when making skin care purchases.

Deciphering the Small Print

The information label on your skin care products is there because the law requires a comprehensive and accurate label. As a consumer, you are entitled to know exactly what ingredients are included in the products you purchase.

The label on your skin care products, by law, must list all ingredients in the product, with the exception of any ingredient that is less than 1 percent of the product. Since 1994, manufacturers have been required to use standardized names for ingredients. International guidelines require that, in addition to the Latin botanical names of plant-derived ingredients, the manufacturers must also include the common names. An example would be "symphytum officinale (comfrey extract)."

The ingredients are listed in descending order. The product contains more of the first ingredient listed than the second, and so on down the entire list of ingredients.

These guidelines protect you, the consumer. You can rest assured that your products don't contain mystery ingredients that could be harmful. And, of equal importance, you can choose to avoid products containing ingredients that may give you an allergic reaction.

The only disappointing aspect of these guidelines is that the manufacturer can list a generalized ingredient, such as "fragrance," without specifying what that fragrance contains. In all fairness, though, some skin products would be quite unappealing without fragrance. They simply don't smell far less than inviting—they smell terrible. A small amount of fragrance makes the product more pleasant to use. But we'd still like to know what specifically is in that fragrance.

> **CAUTION**
> **Wrinkle Guard**
>
> Often the ingredient list is not actually printed on the bottle or jar, but rather on the product box or packaging. Instead of immediately discarding the packaging and its ingredients list, save it just in case you have a bad reaction to the product or simply want to know exactly what you're putting on your skin.

> **Skin-spiration**
>
> Don't be concerned if the first ingredient listed on your skin care products is water. It simply means that all of the hard-working ingredients are in an aqueous, or water-based, solution. Without the water, the product couldn't be formulated.

Cosmeceuticals

Skin care has become much more scientific—and therefore effective—in recent years with the introduction of cosmeceuticals into skin care products. In some ways, the myth of a "miracle in a jar" is no longer a total fantasy.

Cosmeceuticals not only prevent skin damage such as wrinkles, they can also help repair already damaged skin. They help rebuild collagen and elastin. They also reduce irritation. Antioxidants are one example of a cosmeceutical. Antioxidants help prevent skin damage by neutralizing *free radicals* that can damage the skin.

Here's a partial list of cosmeceuticals used widely in skin care products:

- Vitamin A derivatives, such as Retinol
- All vitamins, including A, C, E, and the B vitamins
- Chemical exfoliators (AHAs and BHAs)
- Enzyme exfoliators
- *DMAE* (dimethylaminoethanol)
- Alpha lipoic acid
- Skin lighteners
- Antioxidants
- Pentapeptides

Cosmeceuticals are not the same as pharma-ceuticals, which are prescription-only medications. Popular skin care prescriptions are Retin-A, which is a vitamin A derivative, and hydroquinone, which is a skin lightener. We'll talk more about pharmaceuticals for skin care in Chapter 28.

Clarifying Words

Free radicals are highly active chemicals in the body. They're created from many metabolic processes and also from inflammation and sun damage. They contain one or more unpaired electrons and scavenge, or steal, electrons from other molecules, thus damaging those molecules. In terms of your skin, free radicals can damage collagen and elastin. **DMAE** is dimethylamin-oethanol, a powerful antioxidant which occurs naturally in fish and fish oil. It's used for treatment of attention deficit disorder, dementia, mood disorders, and to improve vision. DMAE is beneficial in reversing the effects of skin aging, such as wrinkles and sagging. It stimulates the muscles to contract and tighten under your skin. DMAE is used both topically and internally.

As noted earlier, the difference between a cosmeceutical and a cosmetic is that cosmetics don't cause the skin to actually change, but cosmeceuticals do. Cosmetics do penetrate the skin, and although they aren't active ingredients, they can be wonderful for the skin. Ingredients such as mineral oil, petrolatum, glycerine, and propylene glycol are considered to be cosmetics.

Body of Knowledge

In recent years, propylene glycol has gained a bad, and unwarranted, reputation. In skin care products, it's a humectant and helps attract water to the skin. Propylene glycol is also used in industrial-strength antifreeze and can be caustic in 100 percent concentrations. But the very small amount used in skin care products is actually beneficial for your skin and isn't irritating. It's made with pure pharmaceutical grade propylene glycol, which is quite different from what's used in your car's radiator. So you don't need to be concerned about any rumors you've heard.

Categories of Ingredients

In any skin care product, many different types of ingredients blend together to produce wonderful and effective concoctions. Individual ingredients work synergistically with all the other ingredients to produce a result. The effect is like a symphony. Just as a favorite concerto or musical composition can't be played with only one instrument, so too an effective skin care product may require many ingredients.

There are thousands of ingredients that can be used in skin care products. We won't list them all in this book, but we will list the categories of ingredients. If you want to learn about specific ingredients, you can purchase an ingredient glossary at most bookstores.

Here are the functional groups of ingredients used in skin care products. As you read through an ingredient list, you'll find these groups of products:

◆ Abrasives. These are exfoliating scrubs and are classified as cosmetics. Includes polyurethane or silicone beads, finely ground corn meal, ground walnut husks, and oatmeal.

◆ Adjusters. Adjusters are cosmetics used to adjust the physical attributes of the product. Some are used to adjust the pH balance, other are used to thicken or thin the products. Includes beeswax, SD alcohol, carbamer 40, and paraffin.

◆ Anti-acne ingredients. These cosmeceuticals can kill off p. acne, the bacteria that causes acne. Includes sulfur, benzoyl peroxide, tea tree oil, camphor, sulfur, and salicylic acid.

- Anti-inflammatories. These cosmeceuticals reduce inflammation in damaged skin. Includes vitamins, aloe, chamomile, grape-seed extract, and raspberry leaf. Oatmeal masks, which contain beta-glucans, are also anti-inflammatories.

- Antioxidants. Cosmeceuticals that are used as both preservatives and as skin treatments. The antioxidants neutralize the free radicals that occur naturally on the skin. They can reduce sun damage and reduce skin aging. Antioxidants include vitamins A, D, and E, plus alpha lipoic acid.

- Alcohols. Alcohols are used primarily in toners for oily skin. SD alcohol is used as a thinning agent for skin products, and it also helps remove oil from the skin, so it can be beneficial for people with oily skin. SD alcohol is noncomedogenic and *antiseptic*. Isopropyl alcohol is drying and *comedogenic*. Avoid using isopropyl alcohol. Benzyl alcohol is useful as an anti-inflammatory on skin care products.

Clarifying Words

A product is **antiseptic** if it inhibits the growth and reproduction of disease-causing microorganisms. Alcohol is antiseptic. **Comedogenic** means that a product promotes clogged pores, which lead to whiteheads, blackheads, and breakouts. An **emulsifier** is a substance that helps keep oils and liquids in suspension to prevent separation of the ingredients. Without the benefits of emulsifiers, products would separate and couldn't clean your face.

- Dyes. These cosmetics have no functional purpose in the skin care product. They give the product an appealing color and are used for their aesthetic value.

- Emollients. Cosmetics that give the product slip and slide. They're present in most skin care products. They prevent moisture in the skin from evaporating and can help prevent skin from becoming dry. Emollients include silicone, mineral oil, petrolatum, lanolin, hyaluronic acid, and shea butter. Tocopherol, also known as vitamin E, can be used both as an emollient and as an antioxidant, which is a cosmeceutical.

- *Emulsifiers.* Emulsifiers are cosmetics used to put oil into solution, so emulsifiers are included in skin care products that have both water-based ingredients and oil-based ingredients. Cleansers often contain emulsifiers that are detergents or surfactants, such as sodium laurel sulfate or polysorbate 20, which give a foaming action to the product that helps "capture" oils and remove them from the skin. Bar soap is an emulsifier, as are lotion cleansers.

◆ Enzymes. Usually derived from plants, such as papaya, pineapple, and pumpkin, they're used as exfoliants and are considered to be cosmeceuticals. They "digest" the dead skin cells and waste products from the surface of the skin.

◆ Fragrance. A cosmetic used to mask the odor of a skin care product. Designer fragrances are often included in European skin care products as part of a signature fragrance line. Most cosmetic and skin care labels simply list "fragrance" in the ingredient list as fragrance and don't give details or specifics.

◆ Herbs. Numerous herbs are used to change skin in a variety of ways, making them cosmeceuticals. For example, chamomile soothes, while green tea is calming and functions as an antioxidant. Comfrey relieves pain, reduces redness, and speeds the healing of wounds. Rose is naturally fragrant, refines pores, and serves as a humectant. You might be allergic to certain herbs, so use caution with herbal skin preparations. Also be aware that some herbs can interact with prescription medications. For example, St. John's Wort can interfere with antidepressant medications.

◆ Humectants. Cosmetics that are used to draw moisture to the skin. Glycerine, honey, urea, propylene glycol, NAPCA, hyaluronic acid, lactic acid, witch hazel, and amino acids are examples of humectants.

◆ Occlusives. Cosmetics used to keep moisture in the skin. Silicones, petrolatum, zinc oxide, titanium dioxide, and mineral oil are all occlusives. Notice, though, that zinc oxide and titanium dioxide are also used as sunscreens, and that mineral oil and silicone are also emollients.

◆ Preservatives and stabilizers. These are cosmetics necessary to extend the shelf life of the products and to keep them from becoming breeding grounds for microorganisms. Hopefully, they are neutral to the skin's functioning. Included in this category are parabens and polysorbate 80.

◆ Skin lighteners. Cosmeceuticals included in skin products specifically marketed as skin lighteners. They include licorice, raspberry, mushroom extract, and vitamin C. Hydroquinone is a skin lightener available only by prescription in concentrations higher than 2 percent. A common over-the-counter brand name for hydroquinone is Porcelana.

CAUTION

Wrinkle Guard

If you are using herbs internally or externally, be sure to phone your pharmacist to make sure that they don't interfere with any prescription medications you may be taking.

CAUTION

Wrinkle Guard

Many suntan lotions are now "paba free" because paba can cause contact dermatitis for some people. For those people, paba is highly irritating to the skin.

◆ Sunscreens. Cosmeceuticals used to protect skin from the UVA and UVB rays of the sun. Sun blocks actually physically block the sun's rays. These include zinc oxide and titanium dioxide. Other sunscreens are chemicals that prevent sun penetration, such as avobenzone, paba, ethylhexyl methoxycinnamate, parsol, and ethylhexyl salicylate.

As you can see, the formulations in skin care products can be very complex. Yet it is this very complexity that gives us such terrific products that rebuild and beautify our skin. It's the symphony of ingredients that keeps our skin healthy.

Vitamins as Cosmeceuticals

We've all been told to take our vitamins. Ingesting them orally provides important nutritional benefits. They make us healthier, improve our immune systems, and can ward off disease. Volumes of scientific research validate the power of vitamins for our health.

We also know that it's possible to absorb vitamins through our skin with very beneficial results. Here's a list of vitamins used in skin care products and their benefits.

◆ Vitamin A and its derivatives, such as Retinol, are used to help reverse sun damage and to inhibit collagen and elastin breakdown. Vitamin A reverses *photo aging* and stimulates collagen synthesis. It's even good for acne, because it peels away layers of skin to help clear up blemishes.

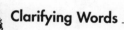

Clarifying Words

Photo aging is a term that refers to skin damage from the sun.

◆ Vitamin E offers a protective barrier for the skin when used topically. Sometimes listed as tocopherol, it helps heal skin wounds and nourishes the skin, allowing it to stretch with ease and helping to prevent stretch marks.

◆ Vitamin C can lighten skin because it's thought to inhibit melanin production. Vitamin C also stimulates formation of collagen. Further research is necessary to understand how it functions for skin lightening.

◆ Vitamin B5, pantothenic acid, aids in the metabolic synthesis of skin lipids and proteins. It also helps the skin to heal. The other B vitamins also nourish the skin.

◆ Vitamin P is a group of bioflavinoids. Strictly speaking, bioflavinoids aren't vitamins, but we list them here because they are a nutrient similar to vitamins.

They include grape seed, ginkgo biloba, and citrus derivatives. These function as antioxidants to eliminate free radicals that can damage skin cells. They also help take redness out of the skin and function as humectants.

So be sure to take your skin vitamins in creams and lotions along with your daily vitamin tablets or capsules. Learn more about which vitamins, minerals, and nutritional supplements taken internally support skin health in Chapter 21.

Naturally Speaking

In recent years, many skin care products claim to be natural. Sounds great. It's easy to assume that all-natural skin care products are safe to use and are actually good for you. But this is seldom the case. Many problems can arise from using completely natural skin care products.

Even the designation "natural" is confusing. Petroleum and mineral oil don't seem natural, but they're by-products of crude oil, which come from natural sources. Crude oil was formed over millions of years from plant and animal materials, which are certainly natural, and organic as well.

CAUTION **Wrinkle Guard** _____

Some consumer advocates are attacking the skin care industry for using ingredients that might be carcinogenic or toxic. We applaud their watchful eyes as being beneficial to everyone's health. However, it's really a problem of proportion. A small amount of lemon oil in a product can be beneficial to your skin. But putting a large amount of lemon oil all over your face would be disastrous because it would burn your face and severely damage your skin. The substances in question by consumer groups are used in small amounts and are highly unlikely to be harmful.

Herbs are natural, and yet some are poisonous or highly irritating to skin. Some herbs are even carcinogenic and toxic. For example, tobacco and tobacco smoke are both. So, natural doesn't necessarily mean safe or even healthy.

Many skin care formulations use natural ingredients, usually combined with other ingredients that make the natural ones even more effective. But using all-natural products can be a serious health and safety concern.

Skin care products that contain only natural ingredients have short shelf lives. They quickly become ineffective, moldy, or filled with dangerous bacteria, often within days of packaging. Virtually all skin care products require some form of preservatives to have a long shelf life, and preservatives contain chemicals. Products that tout themselves as all-natural and chemical-free are therefore highly risky.

If you are determined to only use natural products, be sure to read the labels carefully and be prepared to manage the short shelf life by discarding the products regularly.

> **CAUTION**
>
> ### Wrinkle Guard _____
>
> Andrea wanted to find a new skin care line that would be gentler to her skin. A friend recommended she try an upscale and expensive all-natural line. As soon as her beginner kit arrived, Andrea washed, toned, and moisturized her skin. Within three minutes, her face began to burn and sting, becoming red and inflamed. Ouch. Even totally natural products can cause inflammation and allergic reactions.

Ingredients to Avoid

Today, ingredients in skin care products are thoroughly tested for safety. Use the products as recommended on the package. Discard them at the expiration date, if there is one. It's that simple.

Even though the products are tested and considered safe, that doesn't mean that all products will work for all skin types, or that all products will work well for you. If you experience inflammation, irritation, itching, or redness, stop using the product immediately. Most likely you are sensitive or allergic to the product.

> **Body of Knowledge**
>
> Lanolin is an emollient in skin care products. But it's had a questionable reputation as a skin care ingredient because it was thought to be an allergen and carcinogen. That was before the lanolin producers stopped using pesticides when processing the wool. Recent studies show that only 1.7 percent of the population is allergic to lanolin. If you like the results you get when using lanolin in skin products, then by all means, keep using it. If not, skip it. However, you should never use lanolin on open sores, such as active acne and eczema.

Read the label carefully to make sure the product doesn't contain anything you're allergic to. If it does, don't purchase it. Today, most stores will accept returned skin care products and refund your money, so if you get an unexpected bad reaction, go ahead and return the product.

Some ingredients are comedogenic, meaning they can cause blackheads and white-heads. The products are highly occlusive and prevent your skin's natural oils from flowing to the surface of the skin through the pores. These ingredients include iso-propyl myrastate and cocoa butter. That said, cocoa butter as an ingredient in hand cream can be wonderful. All lipsticks are comedogenic, but you can use them because they are applied to the lips and lips don't get blackheads. However, the skin around them does, so make sure comedogenic products are only applied to the areas they're designed for.

You may want to avoid any product that is highly fragranced if you are sensitive to perfumes. The same applies to dyes. But, overall, just use common sense. If a product doesn't work for you or causes a bad reaction, don't use it.

The Least You Need to Know

- Finding the right product for you means learning to read the labels.
- Cosmeceuticals, unlike cosmetics, actually alter the skin to repair damage and rejuvenate the skin.
- Many types of ingredients are used in skin care products.
- Vitamins work on and in the surface of the skin for protection, repair, and renovation.
- Avoid using products that contain ingredients to which you are allergic or sensitive.

Chapter 9

Becoming a Smart Skin Care Shopper

In This Chapter

- ◆ Setting a budget for skin care
- ◆ Behind the scenes of cosmetics marketing
- ◆ Getting the sales assistance you need
- ◆ Limited brand loyalty

Purchasing skin care products can be overwhelming. It seems like there's an endless variety of products and brands, and we're constantly barraged by advertising and salespeople pushing their products on us. Every brand claims to be the absolute best. Manufacturers state they have research that shows their skin products are wonderful, effective, and well worth the money, but how can you verify that it's true?

The money you spend on skin care is well worth it when you obtain the results you want. Many excellent skin care products cost only pennies a day, others are far more expensive. You can find functional products in every price range. You can purchase your products from exclusive spas and clinics, from up-scale department stores, and at the discount chains and still receive good value and better skin.

In this chapter, we show both men and women how to shop for skin care products. We'll share some trade secrets and give you courage and confidence to purchase skin care products that meet the needs of your skin type, as well as the needs of your budget.

It's Your Decision

Unfortunately, we can't tell you which brand to use. We wish it could be that simple. We would be glad to tell you if we could know your acceptable price range, your skin type, your need for convenience, your lifestyle, and your personal and private belief systems about your skin, but that's obviously not possible. The fact is that everyone's needs are unique.

What we can do is guide you in learning more about yourself and your purchasing needs. Plus, we can alert you to the marketing tools and techniques used by the skin care companies to encourage you to buy. Then you can go to the store forewarned and forearmed.

You can even make it fun to shop for skin care products. Consider it a luxury to be able to walk into a store and know your way around. Once you know what to look for, you'll be happy with your purchases.

Pick a Price Point

You don't need to overspend to have great skin. You can improve your skin by using the skin care products of virtually any brand. So, when starting the process of selecting skin care products, your first consideration needs to be money.

Body of Knowledge
Perhaps you've heard that most of the cost of skin care products is in the promotion and packaging and that the ingredients cost mere pennies. This isn't necessarily so. Today's most popular cosmeceutical ingredients such as sea whip, l-ascorbic acid (Vitamin C), and green tea are expensive. Many cosmeceuticals are patented and that also adds to their cost.

The start-up cost of a good skin care system can range from $24.00 on up to $100.00. That buys you the basics: cleanser, toner, moisturizer, and exfoliant. Expect your initial products to last three months. Then you'll replace them as needed. You can always add to the basics later with such products as eye creams, neck creams, and masks. On an ongoing basis, you can expect to pay anywhere from $10.00 to $100.00 per month for product. Of course, there are plenty of ways to spend more, but you don't need to.

We'd all like to have an unlimited budget for skin care and be able to enjoy all the luxuries, like monthly facials, chemical peels, and extravagant designer cosmetics with fancy packaging. But few of us can truly afford these things on a regular basis. So figure out your monthly skin care allowance and stick to it.

You can be faithful to your budget because today's skin care products all offer similar ingredients at all price levels. They also offer similar proof of efficacy in terms of research studies. In many cases, the ingredients are virtually identical, but with higher-priced products you're also paying for the sales consultant's commission, rental of counter space in the department store, high-priced advertising in fashion magazines and on television, and elegant packaging.

What's Convenient for You

In our hectic and overly busy world, convenience can be a significant factor in skin care. You should expect to purchase at least one of your three basics—cleanser, toner, and moisturizer—every month or two. Most likely, you'll use up the cleanser first. Here are some questions to ask yourself:

- Do I have time to travel to the store for each purchase? If not, will a sales consultant mail the products directly to my home or office and charge my credit card?

- Would I prefer to purchase my skin care products at the grocery store when I do my regular shopping?

- Is it easiest for me to purchase online?

- Do I prefer to bypass the stores and purchase from a friend, such as a Mary Kay Cosmetics consultant?

- Is it worth it to me to make a special trip to the store to purchase routine skin care products?

- Is it a treat for me to go to the store to purchase skin care products?

- Is it convenient for me to purchase my products at a salon or clinic when I go there for regular appointments?

Select your purchasing methods based on what fits into your schedule and lifestyle. We have personally come to greatly appreciate Internet shopping and sales consultants who mail products.

Who Owns What

Upscale cosmetic giants typically own both designer brands and drugstore brands. It's often the case that products from the same manufacturer are sold with different names and prices. Often the product formulations are different and sometimes they are quite similar. Here are some examples, with brands ranked most expensive to least.

- Estee Lauder owns Crème de la Mer, Stila, Bobbie Brown, Estee Lauder, Prescriptives, Origins, MAC, Aveda, Clinique, and Jane.

- L'Oreal owns BioMedic, Biotherm, Lancôme, and Maybelline.

- Proctor & Gamble owns Cover Girl and Oil of Olay.

- Johnson & Johnson owns Aveeno, Neutrogena, and Clean & Clear.

- Revlon owns Revlon, Almay, and Max Factor.

Since a small number of companies own a large number of brands, you can use this to your advantage. This knowledge makes you more powerful as a consumer. Choose a company with a quality that you like and then choose the brand that fits your budget.

Of course, there are many more cosmetic brands than the ones listed above. If you include all the private-label brands used in spas, salons, and skin care studios there are thousands.

Your job is basically to find one brand that fits your budget and works well for your daily skin ritual of cleansing, toning, and moisturizing. For other skin care products, such as hand cream and exfoliators, you can stay with your skin care brand or find other products from other brands.

You can have great-looking skin by shopping at the department stores, shopping at the high-end specialty stores, or by shopping at Wal-Mart. Don't feel inferior if you are on a limited budget. There's no reason for your face to reflect it.

A Brand for Your Daily Skin Ritual

Finding a *skin care line* or brand that works well for your skin is basically hit and miss. You can certainly gather information from friends, magazines, and *Consumer Reports*, but no one can tell you what lines will work best on your skin. You may want to consider using the skin care system your mother used. Since you inherited some of the qualities of her skin, this may be a good place to look first. Skin care lines change their formulations every two or three years so your mother's line may or may not work as well for you. Be sure to shop at the stores that offer skin care products in your price range.

The bottom line on selecting a brand is this: The only way to find out if a skin care line works for your skin is to use the products for about three weeks. Then you can judge the result for yourself.

When you purchase products from a skin care line, ask the sales consultant if you can return the products if they don't work for you. If the sales consultant says no refunds, move to another counter. This whole process can be difficult enough without your needing to keep investing in products that don't work. Often, a line will give you samples to try. This gets you off the hook for having to return merchandise and saves the skin care line money as well.

For the sake of your skin, and to get the very best results, use a cleanser, toner, and moisturizer from the same skin care line. These products are scientifically formulated in the laboratory to work *synergistically*. Used together, the three products normalize your skin's pH (acid/alkaline) balance, provide proper skin hydration, and assure that the moisturizer is effective. If you substitute another product, you'll likely be disappointed.

Clarifying Words

A **skin care line** is a term referring to a brand's skin care products. This is a common usage in the skin care industry and at department store sales counters. **Synergistically** means that the combined interaction of the three products—cleanser, toner, and moisturizer—is greater than the sum of their effects individually.

When it comes to other skin care products, such as exfoliators, shaving gels, eye cream, and hand cream, feel free to purchase products from any line. You don't need to be faithful to a skin care line for anything but the three basics.

Also be sure to use the same products every day. Don't use one product line one day, and another the next. In a sense, this confuses your skin and it won't want to behave.

Changing Skin Care Lines

It's unlikely that you'll stay with the same products throughout your life. Youthful skin has different needs than skin over 30, 40, or 50. As your skin changes, expect to change your skin care products. Many skin care lines have different formulations to suit different kinds of skin and skin ages. You may be able to shift products within a line, or you may need to find a new line altogether.

Here are some reasons you may want to change skin care lines:

◆ You have a skin condition that requires special treatment. These conditions are described in Part 4. Included are congestion, dehydration, sun damage, and rosacea.

◆ You're no longer satisfied with your skin and want to try something new.

◆ You want to use the cosmeceuticals you've read about.

◆ You're making more money and want to use more expensive products.

◆ You want to save money and know you can still get great skin results for less money.

◆ Your skin has matured and you need more nourishing skin care products.

◆ You want to use the skin care system recommended by a skin care technician or friend.

◆ For no good reason at all—you just want a change.

Follow the same skin care selection guidelines when you are making your initial purchase or when you are changing lines.

Marketing a Brand

When you understand how skin care lines market to consumers, you can make a better buying decision. The first thing to realize is that skin care companies know how to get your business. They know your buying emotions and your timing. They invest many millions in target marketing to you, the skin care consumer.

Here's what advertisers do to capture your interest:

◆ Advertise with glamorous full-page ads in magazines, often with pictures of celebrity movie stars or famous high-fashion models.

◆ Use gorgeous young models or movie stars in ads, implying that you can look as good and live as elegantly if you purchase their products.

◆ Cite "research" results that show the effectiveness of their products. The studies aren't published in scientific journals or available to the consumer, nor are they *double-blind* studies. The research was paid for by the company and may be biased.

◆ Encourage sales of specific brands through commissions. Department stores and salons usually

Clarifying Words

A **double-blind** research study uses a control group to validate a study's results. One group uses the product, one group doesn't. Neither group nor the professionals administering the study know which group is using the product or which group isn't. This is essential to truly scientific studies. Cosmetic companies typically don't follow this procedure, so their acclaimed results are not as scientifically valid.

pay their sales consultants commissions and assign them sales quotas, so they have a vested interest in making the sale. This isn't always the case, but it's standard. You can always ask the sales consultant if he or she is paid on commission.

- **Pay the stores for location.** Yes, the cosmetic brand that has the counter closest to the front of the department store or closest to the main aisle pays extra for the most visible location. In grocery stores and discount chains, brands sometimes pay to have their products placed at eye level, so you notice them first.

- **Connect a theme with their brand.** Perhaps you think of Aveda or Origins as all-natural lines because of how the product is presented. Clinique is positioned as scientific—so much so that the sales consultants wear lab coats. Almay is positioned as nonallergenic. The theme may or may not be accurate.

- **Associate fashion designers with the line.** Chanel, Dior, and Yves Saint Laurent are skin care lines that imply they were designed by a fashion designer. They weren't, but the line is sometimes owned by a fashion house. Designer lines are among the most expensive and often the most highly fragranced.

- **Never go on sale.** There are a few exceptions, but typically you won't get a price break—ever.

- **Promote gifts with purchases.** This only *seems* like a sale. By spending a certain minimum amount, such as $20, you receive a goodie bag filled with cosmetics and samples. It makes us feel like we've received a bonus prize, and the goodie bags are fun. However, we also just spent $20 or more. Gifts with purchase get consumers who want to spend money into the stores.

- **Package beautifully.** Admittedly, there's terrific allure in having a beautiful package. It makes the product emotionally satisfying because we associate the quality of the product with the beauty of the packaging design. Practically speaking, the elegant packaging adds nothing to the product's worth, but it does add to your cost. Even knowing that, it's still hard to resist an interestingly shaped bottle and a sleek label.

- **Offer on-the-spot makeovers.** You become the "guppy" in a goldfish bowl as other customers view your transformation. The brand's hope is that you'll feel obliged to purchase everything the consultant applied to your face, while also turning you into a free billboard for his or her products.

- **Bring in the celebrity creator of the line or a special makeup artist.** You may even be asked to schedule a time slot for your makeover. You'll also be expected to purchase lots of product. However, this can be a great opportunity to get a new and updated look and to learn about new treatment products.

♦ Highlight exclusive distribution. Some skin care products are available only through infomercials, some only at a medical skin care clinic. For some consumers, the notion of exclusive means better or best. Practically speaking, exclusive only means that you may have to jump through hoops and spend more to purchase these products.

♦ Target market to ethnic groups, such as blacks and Hispanics. We applaud this from the point of view that their color palates for foundations, lipsticks, eye shadows, and cheek colors are designed to work with a wide variety of ethnic skin tones.

CAUTION

Wrinkle Guard

Many skin care boutiques, spas, and salons carry private-label skin care products. Some claim the products are developed and formulated by the owners. Sometimes this is true, but other times the owners have merely selected from a wide array of formulations available for private label. Several large companies do the manufacturing and formulation, and the owner supplies the name and label.

Skin-spiration

The top-selling skin care line in the United States is Mary Kay, ahead of any department store or drug store brand. Mary Kay associates sell directly to the consumer through home parties. Their sales associates number in the hundreds of thousands. Mary Kay offers relatively inexpensive yet effective skin care products that contain up-to-date cosmeceutical treatments.

Spas and skin care boutiques use some of the same marketing techniques as the department stores. They offer skin treatments and then recommend skin care products specifically for your skin type. Yes, they make a profit on the products, and that's fine. Just know that you can say yes or no based on budget, convenience, and your feelings about the product. Don't let pressure and sales tactics determine your skin care!

By understanding the marketing tactics of skin care lines, you can choose to purchase or not purchase, but you won't be easily seduced into buying products that you don't need, can't use, and will regret spending money on before you enter your driveway.

The Good Side

Cosmetic companies want your business. There's a strong upside to all this. Because they want you as a customer, cosmetics companies really are trying to offer products that help you realize your dreams of radiant and healthy skin.

Because of this, sales consultants are well trained by manufacturers in skin and skin care, and they understand the ins and outs of their product offerings. They know that if you're satisfied with their skin care products, you'll keep purchasing them. You can phone them with your questions, and, at the time of purchase, receive instruction in how to specifically use the products.

Some drugstores now have a designated sales consultant in the skin care and cosmetics area. This person is knowledgeable about the products on the shelves and can answer your questions. We applaud drugstores for providing this valuable service.

If the products you purchase don't perform as you expect, sales consultants can give you advice and make recommendations. They're usually quite experienced in solving skin care problems and can add a dose of common sense when needed.

Just for Men

Some advanced skin care companies are leading edge. They recognize that men want to have great-looking skin, too. They also know that few men will stand in front of a department store cosmetic counter and ask for advice. After all, men are famous for not asking for directions. Why would they willingly stand in the women's section of a store asking for advice?

Along comes the men's section. You can often find men's skin care products in the men's perfume and cologne section of department stores. You can also purchase men's lines online.

Are men's products different than women's? Essentially, no. The five skin types are the same for both men and women, and the same products work for men and women. If there's any difference at all, it's only skin deep—the packaging comes in masculine colors and more angular designs. Fragrances may seem more "manly."

Men can shop for men's skin care products, or men can purchase the same products women use. It depends on your preference, stamina, and courage. But, by all means, purchase and use the products you need to put your best face forward.

The Deciding Factor

Personal preference is characterized by how you think of yourself and how you perceive a skin care line. All of the marketing research in the world can't accurately predict how you personally will make a buying decision.

Your beliefs about your skin, your social status, and your lifestyle dictate your choices. For example, some women will sacrifice the grocery budget to purchase a $75 jar of moisturizer. Some women eagerly look forward to the day when their income increases enough to comfortably purchase department store or designer skin care lines.

Men may borrow skin care products from their wives or friends rather than been seen purchasing products at the store. They think that wouldn't be masculine. On the other hand, some men get regular facials at a skin care salon.

Many men and some women don't want to mess with their skin and can't imagine buying much more than the mere basics plus lip balm.

Respect your belief system. Whatever you do for your skin, it needs to fit you and who you are. Otherwise, you'll ultimately be disappointed.

Discontinued Products

In the normal course of doing business, skin care companies discontinue products and replace them with others. This is especially upsetting if you've become attached to a certain product. Here are a couple of suggestions for filling this void in your life:

- Try the "replacement" product. In many cases, new versions of products contain revamped formulations that may work even better for your skin.

- Buy up all the stock of a discontinued product that you can find. Store it in the refrigerator to extend its shelf life. One of the authors purchased six of the same eye shadow sets when the product was discontinued. Three years later, it still seems like it was a good decision, and with some luck the eye shadows may last 10 more years.

- Go online and check eBay and wholesale sites to find the item. We did this with a discontinued aromatherapy body lotion and found about 10 tubes available for purchase.

If none of these work, take heart. With the wide array of available products on the market, you can find skin care happiness and contentment with other products. In fact, you'll probably find a new product that you'll like even more than the one that was discontinued.

The Least You Need to Know

- Shopping for the right skin care products begins with understanding your own needs and budget.

- Enjoy all the "glamour" associated with skin care, but make your buying decision based on practical concerns.

- Being aware of the marketing practices of skin care manufacturers will help you make a wise purchase.

- Sales consultants offer knowledge and experience that can help you use their products successfully.

- Men can use the same skin care products as women, or choose products specifically aimed at men, but both will be equally effective.

Chapter 10

Laying the Foundation

In This Chapter

- The benefits of foundation
- What foundation can (and can't) do for your skin
- Making your color selection
- Properly applying foundation and concealer

After cleansing, toning, and moisturizing, you can apply a light veil of color. A little color on your face adds a finishing touch to your skin. If you've stayed faithful to your daily routine for a while, then your skin is healthier and glowing, and color shows off the daily care you've taken.

Color comes in many forms, from a barely there tinted moisturizer to color with more substantial coverage, as in pancake makeup. The most up-to-date look is light, and the heavier and thicker foundations are best reserved for professional photography and stage and television makeup. Yes, even pancake makeup can be applied lightly.

Color, or foundation, is now considered to be a skin treatment, but an optional one. Color offers additional sun protection, can enhance your moisturizer's effectiveness, or can absorb your skin's natural oil secretions to give you a more matte look.

In addition to health benefits, a little color can make you feel more polished, boost your self-esteem, and give you the confidence to face the world at large.

Protecting Your Skin

Today's color, or foundation (we use the words interchangeably in this chapter), is virtually revolutionary in its benefits to your skin. Once upon a time, foundation was considered to be a cover-up and a way to hide wrinkles and blemishes. Color palettes were often way too pink or way too orange to blend with anyone's natural coloring, and people of color weren't able to purchase a foundation that even came close to matching their individual skin tones.

All that has changed, and we applaud the changes. The biggest difference is that color or foundation these days is actually good for your skin, offers you valuable protection from pollution and the sun, and helps you balance oily and dry skin. Foundation is now formulated to make your skin healthier and to encourage your skin to radiate.

Pollution Guard

It happens if you live in a big city, or a small town. It happens when you drive your car. It happens if you work in a building with heating and air-conditioning. And it happens if you work in a factory or in a hair salon. Every day, and in many ways, your exposed skin is bombarded with pollutants. And, unfortunately, the most exposed parts of your body are your face and hands.

Some pollution shows up as soot, dust, and visible particulates. Other pollutants are minuscule, but even when you can't see them, pollutants are depositing free radicals on your skin. These free radicals damage your skin and create wrinkles, bumps, irritation, and inflammation. So, of course, you want a way to keep those pollutants away from direct contact with your skin.

For this purpose, moisturizer alone isn't enough. Instead, you need a veil that keeps your skin clean and clear, a veil that you can wash every night, confident that most of the pollutants you've encountered are going straight down the drain.

The answer? A thin layer of color or foundation. The pollutants get "captured" by your foundation. That's not to say that foundation captures all forms of pollutants that can damage skin. We wish it were so. But foundation does add a protective layer, and because you want the best for your skin, every little bit helps.

Sun Barrier

In addition to staving off some of the damage from pollution, foundations now come with sunscreen added. The sunscreen is usually a sun block that acts as a physical barrier, preventing the sun's rays from penetrating your skin. The rays get reflected off the surface of your foundation.

The sun block ingredients are usually zinc oxide and/or titanium oxide. These protect against both UVA and UVB rays. For the best sunscreen protection, you should still use a sunscreen before applying your foundation. Use a foundation with a sunscreen of SPF 15 or higher. A foundation rated less than SPF 15 is best left for evening wear.

The SPF—sun protection factor—of sunscreen is not cumulative. So if your moisturizer has an SPF of 15 and your foundation has an SPF of 15, you don't get sun protection of an SPF of 30 by applying both. Your protection *is* greater than 15, but we can't tell you exactly how much more because various products interact differently. So, to be on the safe side, assume you still have a sun protection factor of 15 and use other sunscreens accordingly. SPF and the use of sunscreens are discussed in detail in Chapter 16.

Skin-spiration

Perhaps you remember when the lifeguards at the pool or the beach slathered their noses with a bright white cream. Although it may have looked silly, they were using zinc oxide as a total sun block. Zinc oxide is naturally bright white, but when it is added to foundations today for sun protection it blends with the more natural color. Just think, now you can give your skin great protection by wearing zinc oxide all over your face and it will look completely natural!

Be sure not to rely on your foundation as your only sunscreen. To use sunscreen correctly, you need to use quite a bit and apply it on every area of your face. We doubt you want to use that much foundation. And, if your foundation gets smeared—while you're talking on the phone and it's cradled between your shoulder and cheek, for example—you'll lose sunscreen protection in that area.

Mineral makeup is both an excellent foundation and sunscreen. The very finely powdered minerals include zinc oxide and titanium dioxide. Titanium dioxide is also a natural anti-inflammatory. Because the makeup is a powder, it doesn't contain any creams, lotions, or emollients that can cause breakouts or allergic reactions. Mineral makeup gives your skin a radiant glow while optically masking blemishes and darker pigmentation. The sunscreen protection of the various brands can range from SPF 15 to 20. Just brush on, look radiant, and have instant long-lasting, water-resistant sun protection.

Balancing Oil and Dryness

Today's foundations give your cleanser, toner, and moisturizer a little help by complementing their effectiveness. If you have skin with an excess of oil, as in oily or acne-type skin, you can purchase oil-free foundations. You can even go one step further and purchase oil-absorbing foundations that contain *microsponges*.

Don't worry, no one ground up a kitchen sponge and put the shreds into your foundation. Instead, the microsponges are sterile oxylate polymers, basically a form of plastic that can absorb up to four times their weight in sebum. Very clever, huh?

Some foundations are formulated specifically for someone with drier skin, who wears a richer moisturizer. This could be a person with sensitive-type skin or a person with surface dryness. You can choose from two kinds of foundations. The first is occlusive and prevents moisture loss. The second contains emollients and humectants that add additional moisture to the skin. How do you know which is which? Ask your sales consultant. We'll talk more about that in a moment when we discuss purchasing foundation.

Color Is Optional

Using color or foundation is totally optional. You don't need to wear it to have healthy and clear skin. However, if you are avoiding foundation because of a long-standing bias, you might want to reconsider.

You may be avoiding foundation because you already have great skin, you like your skin tone, or you want the natural look. For some women, not needing or wearing foundation is a sort of status symbol. They view foundation as a product exclusively for people with skin problems to hide.

If you are at all open to trying color, consider the protection and treatment aspects before you choose to pass it by. If you're unhappy with the idea of thick, visible makeup, take a look at what's currently on the market. Today's formulations are so sheer that some are nearly invisible and they definitely suit the natural look.

Overall, foundation as color can make a big difference in the health of your skin. It's one more way for you to create good skin—treating the outer layer with a protective barrier. In Part 5, you'll learn to create fabulous skin from the inside out through diet and exercise.

What Color Can Do

As a cosmetic, foundation can only do so much. But with today's new technology and formulations, it can do way more than you might think. Here's what you can reasonably expect:

♦ Foundation isn't intended to cover up your face or conceal flaws. Don't use foundation as a mask.

♦ Foundation can even out pigmentation to give your skin a more uniform color and can brighten your complexion.

♦ Foundation creates a polished finish to your skin. Before an artist starts painting on canvas, he or she prepares the canvas with a thin coat of gesso. The gesso makes the canvas smoother and fills in some of the rougher texture. Foundation, in a sense, does the same thing as gesso—it gives your skin a smoother finish.

♦ Foundation can't correct blemishes, but it can diminish their appearance. However, it can make your skin appear *less* blemished. This means that, at first glance, blemishes may not be noticeable, but foundation is not a concealer. If you have serious blemishes to cover up, first use a concealer, then apply foundation.

♦ Foundation can't cover up dents and pockmarks, nor can it cover up birthmarks and extreme pigmentation areas. However, you can purchase camouflage makeup as a cover-up. With the proper application, you'll look great.

♦ Foundation can help cover up rosacea and broken capillaries.

♦ If you use other cosmetics, such as blush and eye makeup, foundation gives you a base upon which to paint. It actually makes the other products work better and go on evenly and smoothly.

Foundation can give you the appearance of great-looking skin as you rebuild your skin's health. This will enhance your self-esteem and give you the confidence you desire.

CAUTION

Wrinkle Guard _____

At the end of a late night out on the town, it's easy to skip cleansing your face. Don't! This is when your skin needs cleansing the most. If you use foundation, you must wash your face every evening. Evening means anytime from late afternoon until just before bed. After all, you want to flush the daily buildup of toxins and pollutants down the drain.

Types of Foundation

There are hundreds of different kinds of foundations, with new ones available almost weekly. A new one has arrived at the department stores as we write this book—a light beam on the skin supposedly determines the best shade for every skin. With new technology such as this constantly emerging, the art and science of foundations seems to be perpetually evolving.

Healthy skin is supposed to look dewy, moist, and plump. But not everyone favors that look, especially if they have oily or acne-type skin. Foundations can make your skin appear dewy or void of oil. Here are the basic types of foundations:

◆ Sheer tints like pink and apricot offer just a touch of color. They're not skin-toned, but they give a lift to your face. Don't use them as moisturizers. Instead, apply these foundations over your moisturizer.

◆ Tinted moisturizers give a very light, transparent finish. Even though they are labeled as moisturizers, use a standard moisturizer before applying. Otherwise you are applying color directly into your pores, which you definitely don't want to do. As the foundation "moves and migrates" during the day, you could end up looking as if you painted dots on your pores.

◆ Liquid foundations offer a wide variety of coverage and are the most popular. These are made for every skin type. They can be oil-free or moisturizing.

◆ Pancake foundations are rich, creamy formulas that offer more coverage and make the skin appear moist and dewy.

◆ Powder foundations come in a portable compact, don't spill, and can give your skin a powdery matte finish.

◆ Matte foundations mask the appearance of oily skins and often contain oil-absorbing ingredients.

◆ Light-diffusing foundations use light-reflecting particles to camouflage pigmentation and fine wrinkles. They also give your skin an added glow and radiance.

◆ Loose mineral powders are applied with a brush. Many are often packaged in a convenient brush dispenser, They are light-diffusing and give your skin a warm glow and are typically free of allergens and chemicals that can cause irritation.

Skin-spiration

If you have oily skin that appears shiny by midday, use rice blotting papers to blot away the oil. Your face will regain its composure. Rice blotting papers are widely available at drugstores and discount chains.

As you can tell, you have plenty of choices for foundation. Be sure to sample several different types to make sure you purchase the type that works best to you. You may even want to purchase a couple different types for different occasions, such as one with heavier coverage for evenings out and a light-diffusing foundation for the office.

At the Store

Of all the skin care products, foundation is the hardest to buy. You want just the right color in just the right formulation for your skin. It seems exhausting, but don't let it be. You may need to make several trips to multiple stores to find perfection, but with all the choices available, rest assured that you will eventually find the right foundation.

Ideally, you can find a color that matches your skin tone. Skin tones either have a pink undertone or a yellow undertone. If you've had a difficult time finding a foundation that blends well with your skin, most likely, you're using a pink undertone when you need a yellow-base or vice versa. When shopping for foundation, ask the sales consultant to find the undertones that blend best with your skin tone.

Here are some shopping tips:

◆ Start shopping first at the department stores because you can try on the foundation and check right then and there to see if the color works for you.

◆ Ask for help. Tell the sales consultant your skin type and what results you want from a foundation.

◆ When you find a color that looks good indoors under florescent lights, borrow a mirror and walk outside to check the color in natural light. This is a good reason to shop for foundation during the day rather than at night.

◆ Test the color on the front of your cheek where you can see it. Often, sales consultants want to test products on the side of your face near the jaw line. We find it virtually impossible to see that part of our faces clearly in a mirror. Test foundation where you can see it. Don't test for color on your hand or on your neck; test where will you actually apply the foundation.

◆ Ask for samples to take home and use for a couple of days. That way, you'll know for sure if the foundation works for you with regular application. Most sales consultants will fill a small bottle for you. Keep the bottle—you can use it to refill for your handbag or for traveling.

◆ You only need one foundation that works for both day and evening, and you only need one color—the one that matches your skin. The possible exception is using a lighter foundation in winter and a slightly darker one for summer.

◆ Go shopping when you're in a good mood and feel good about your skin. Buying a new foundation is ineffective at mending a broken heart or lightening up your day—that's expecting too much from a bottle!

◆ Purchase any brand that works for you. You don't need to use the same brand that you use to cleanse, tone, and moisturize.

◆ A bottle of foundation should last a long time, as in six months to a year or more. If you are replacing foundation much more frequently than that, you're using way too much. The exception is if you have active acne. In that case, replace your foundation every three to four months to keep it free from bacterial growth.

Skin-spiration

If your basic daily skin care is good and you are cleansing, toning, and moisturizing twice a day, you should have no problem wearing foundation. If you find that your foundation seems to be causing irritation or redness, talk with your sales consultant for advice. If that doesn't work, choose another brand with different ingredients.

◆ If you use a self-tanner on your face, make sure your face is tanned before you shop for foundation. Either that, or use a bronzing powder with a foundation that's your natural skin tone.

◆ If you have dark skin, it's fine to be picky. Don't settle for an OK color—get a *great* color. To find a skin care line that carries foundation for darker skin tones, pick up a copy of a magazine such as *Ebony* or *Black Essence* and check out the advertisements. The same goes for darker skin tones.

◆ It's harder to find the right color of foundation when shopping at a drugstore or discount chain. You can't try on the color or take home a sample. If you try to match a color by comparing the color of the bottles, you could be very disappointed when you get home. The color may not even be close to the same once you try it on. Always ask if you can return the foundation before you buy.

Yes, it takes stamina and perseverance to purchase the best foundation. Sales consultants have seen a huge range of skin types and helped thousands of people with color-matching. Ask for their advice and use it. If you aren't satisfied at one counter, feel free to ask what other lines might have the formulation and color that will meet your needs.

Applying Foundation

Now that you've purchased your foundation, it's time to learn the best ways to apply it. First of all, be sure to cleanse, tone, and moisturize your skin before you apply any color or foundation. By doing this, you set the best backdrop for color application.

Next, put a dime-sized amount of foundation on the back of your nondominant hand. With new formulations, you only need a small amount to cover your face.

With your dominant hand—the one you write with—pick up a sponge and dab lightly into the foundation. A sponge makes a terrific applicator. You get enough color, but not too much. You can easily use the sponge to blend the foundation over your entire face.

Sponges are disposable, so make sure you get the most value from each sponge. Each day, use a new corner until each corner is used up, then discard it. Or use a circular sponge and cut into eighths, using a new side everyday. This will last you 16 days. You can either wash out the sponge for reuse or toss it out.

Don't take a big sponge to your face. The application will be more difficult and you'll end up using way more foundation than you need.

CAUTION

Wrinkle Guard

Don't use your fingers to apply foundation. The oils in your fingertips can break down the formulation and the foundation won't last as long on your face.

To apply, use the sponge to dab a small amount of foundation on the center parts of your face, including your chin, nose, cheeks, and forehead. Dab on only one area at a time, then spread and blend the foundation outward toward the ears, temples, and jaw. Proceed to the next area and continue applying until all areas are covered.

Don't forget your nose or the inner corners of your eyes near the bridge of your nose. Be careful not to apply foundation too close to your hairline, and avoid getting it in your hair. Stop just short of your jaw line and then blend down over the jaw line and feather off lightly down your neck. Don't apply foundation to your neck because the foundation is certain to rub off on your clothing.

Skin-spiration

You no longer need to wear a heavier foundation for evening. Instead, add more intense lipstick, eye makeup, or cheek color for drama.

CAUTION

Wrinkle Guard

Use powder blusher over a powder-based foundation and a cream blush over a cream-based foundation. They'll go on smoother and look more natural.

You need to work rather quickly to get the foundation applied before it dries. As you develop more expertise, you should be able to do your entire face in just a minute or two. If your skin seems to need more than just a dime-sized amount of foundation, you may not be cleansing, toning, and moisturizing correctly. The foundation should easily glide on your skin when it is properly prepared.

Check to make sure that you have blended the foundation completely and that you don't have any streaks. If you do, smooth them out with the sponge. Stand back and admire your handiwork. If you want to add a dusting of powder to set your foundation, now is the time to brush or puff. Next, apply additional makeup, such as eye shadow, blush, or lipstick, as desired.

If you have dark spots or blemishes you want to conceal, read on and learn about the art of using concealer.

Concealer

It's true that foundation isn't intended to cover up your skin. Rather, it's meant to let your skin glow. But what about those times when you really do want to cover up a blemish or disguise dark circles under your eyes?

Enter concealer. This product is specifically designed to be a cover-up. Concealer is waxy and is meant to stay in place. It sits on top of your skin. Be sure to use it sparingly, and only where you need more coverage.

You can use concealer either before or after you apply foundation. Most people use it before, but the choice is up to you. Experiment and find out what works best for you.

Concealer comes in a limited number of colors—usually light, medium, and dark. For darker skin, you'll find more variety. Apply the concealer lightly and sparingly with a sponge applicator or with a small brush. Use a stippling technique to make it look more natural. Stippling is sort of like applying lots of small dots of color that intersect with each other.

Don't apply concealer with your fingers. As with foundation, the oil in your fingertips will alter the formulation and make it less effective, oilier, and less waxy, so the concealer won't stay in place and will tend to migrate.

The Least You Need to Know

◆ Color, or foundation, gives a polished finishing touch to your face that lets your skin shine through.

◆ Selecting a foundation is hard work, so be prepared to spend enough time to find the right shade and brand for you.

◆ Prepare your skin for foundation by cleansing, toning, and moisturizing first.

◆ Apply foundation carefully with a light hand to obtain the glow and radiance you want.

◆ Foundation will not cover up blemishes, and if that is a concern, you may need to use a concealer.

Part 4

Combating Common Skin Conditions

Thank goodness, skin conditions are only temporary. But that doesn't mean you don't want to correct them as quickly as possible. We tell you exactly how to identify and what to do to solve the following skin conditions: acne, congestion and breakouts, rosacea, dehydration, sensitized skin, sun damage, abnormal pigmentation, premature aging, and menopausal skin.

You'll learn the secrets that skin care technicians at spas and salons use to soothe, heal, and comfort troubled skin. You'll obtain information on both natural healing treatments and commercially available solutions. Plus, if your skin starts behaving badly in the future, you can refer to this part of the book to get it back on track.

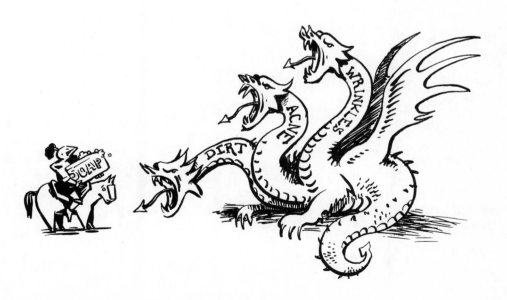

Chapter 11

Dealing with Acne

In This Chapter

- ◆ Fighting acne bacteria
- ◆ Recognizing acne trigger points
- ◆ Changing lifestyles to manage acne
- ◆ Getting help from professionals

Of all the skin conditions and blemishes, one of the most common and most dreaded is acne. Acne can be socially embarrassing and cause you to lose faith in your ability to maintain healthy and clear skin. The good news is that you *can* control acne. You can manage acne so that it becomes inactive and eruptions virtually never occur. With some work, your skin can stay calm and soothed and be free of blemishes.

To get started, you may need some medicinal intervention. And you'll need to develop a "hands-off" approach when you're tempted to pick at an acne eruption. Mastering acne requires making some lifestyle changes, employing excellent skin care habits, and paying attention to diet and exercise.

In this chapter we tell you all about acne—what causes it, how to care for active acne, and how to get acne into an inactive state and keep it there.

The Definition of Acne

Acne is defined as a skin eruption caused by the bacteria propionibacterium acne, or p. acne. P. acne only grows in the skin, not inside the body. If the eruption doesn't have these bacteria present, it isn't acne. As much as those with acne-type skin may not want to hear this, getting acne is part of one's genetic makeup.

Does that mean that if you have acne-type skin you're doomed to a lifetime of active acne outbreak? Not at all. But it does mean that you're more likely to break out than other types.

Even if you have acne-type skin, it's possible that you will never have an eruption. It's also possible that your skin won't erupt until you experience a highly stressful time in your life. This can happen at any age, but if it happens when you're an adult, your condition is known as adult-onset acne.

A person with acne-type skin has body chemistry that's vulnerable to p. acne. This means that the p. acne bacteria can live in and on your skin.

Acne Gets a Grade

You could have anything from mild acne to intense acne. Here are the grades used by skin care technicians. Dermatologists and medical skin-care experts use only three categories, but we want you to be familiar with all of them:

Clarifying Words

A **comedone** is a pore clogged with sebum and dead skin cells. Products that are comedogenic, such as lanolin and petrolatum promote the formation of blackheads and whiteheads.

- ◆ Grade One: Inactive acne. You have no inflammation and your skin feels normal—no points of hurt or pain. You are taking great care of your skin, cleansing, toning, moisturizing, and exfoliating with salicylic acid regularly. No one can tell by looking that you have acne-type skin.

- ◆ Grade Two: Whiteheads and blackheads. Whiteheads are closed *comedones;* blackheads are open comedomes. You may have some small early-stage red bumps under the surface of your skin.

- ◆ Grade Three: Mild eruptions. Your skin is not severely inflamed. Under the surface are closed comedomes with fewer blackheads.

- ◆ Grade Four: Pustules or raised bumps. You have many closed comedones with inflamed pores. They are starting to be both red and white with pus underneath the surface of the skin.

- ◆ Grade Five: Hard nodules. You have cysts under the surface of your skin. They're tender to the touch. They may even hurt. You have both closed and open comedomes.

- ◆ Grade Six: Totally active acne. Everything seems to be happening to your skin at once—whiteheads, blackheads, pustules, papules, cysts. It's painful and hurts to touch your face, which is highly inflamed. Go straight to the doctor.

If you suspect that your skin rates a grade of four or higher, you need to visit a dermatologist about your skin condition. Ask for skin care product recommendations and get information about possible prescription medications that he would advise. Be sure to carefully research the side effects and long-term effects of any prescription medications before you start taking them.

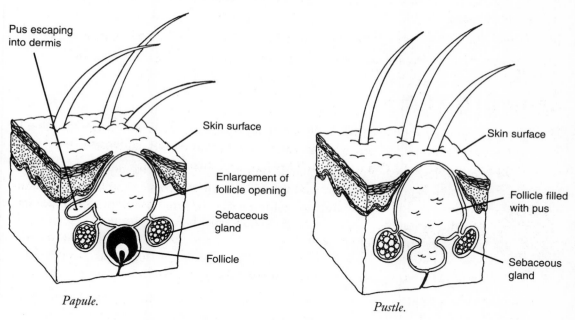

Papule.

Pustle.

Killing Off P. Acne

Now that you know that it is bacteria that causes acne, it simply doesn't make sense to pick or squeeze a bump. Here's why. When you squeeze, you create more inflammation and p. acne lives on inflammation. Also, when you squeeze, you encourage the p. acne to spread under the skin to new areas. One squeeze can trigger lots of new bumps close by. To sum it up, squeezing encourages more acne. The p. acne may like that you squeeze, but you and your skin won't like the results.

Some products are excellent at helping heal your skin and ultimately killing off p. acne bacteria. Here's a list:

◆ Sulfur. Sulfur unclogs pores and removes p. acne bacteria. Also used to reduce inflammation. Over-the-counter acne medications contain sulfur.

> **Body of Knowledge**
>
> Tea tree oil is an essential oil distilled from the leaves of the melaluca plant which is native to Australia. The oil is active against bacteria, viruses, and fungal infections. It's used to aid in healing abscesses, acne, athlete's foot, blisters, burns, cold sores, dandruff, herpes, insect bites, oily skin, rashes, and warts.

◆ Tea tree oil. Tea tree oil kills p. acne and is an ingredient in many acne skin care formulations—cleansers, toners, and moisturizers. Tea tree oil is considered as effective as benzoyl peroxide for killing p. acne bacteria, but it takes longer. However, tea tree oil doesn't cause the redness, irritation, and inflammation that's common with benzoyl peroxide.

◆ Benzoyl peroxide. P. acne can't live in the presence of oxygen. Benzoyl peroxide forms oxygen deep in the pore and the p. acne dies off. Benzoyl peroxide is drying to the skin and can make it peel. Benzoyl peroxide is an active ingredient in many over–the-counter acne products.

◆ Antibiotics. Antibiotics are available only by prescription from your doctor and include tetracycline and erythromycin. It's not advised to use these for an extended period of time because antibiotics have undesirable side effects, such as dehydration of the skin and killing off beneficial intestinal bacteria, which results in yeast-overgrowth infections. You can also build up resistance to the effectiveness of these antibiotics, and antibiotics can interfere with the effectiveness of other medications, such as birth control pills.

◆ Retin-A. This prescription medication is applied topically. It's derived from vitamin A, and it helps prevent the formation of microcomedomes in which the p. acne live and multiply. Retin-A removes the top layers of skin so no oil can be trapped in the pores. Retin-A can be used for longer periods of time. Think of Retin-A as a super-exfoliator. Because Retin-A thins the skin, you need intense sun protection every day because your face is far more susceptible to burning than normal. Also, avoid waxing your upper lip or anywhere on your face when using this product. Wear a hat that shades your face when outdoors.

◆ Accutane. Accutane is a prescription-only medication that's taken internally. Accutane is vitamin A at a very high dose. Use only with severe acne eruptions. Accutane severely dries up mucous membranes and has serious side effects including birth defects and mental disorders. You must sign a consent form before taking the medication. If a woman decides to take Accutane, she needs to provide two negative pregnancy tests and must use two separate effective forms of birth control for the month before starting Accutane. You receive a 30-day supply at a time and will be required to have a monthly blood test to make sure you stay healthy. A national registry is being proposed to track persons who have used this powerful medication for long-term safety studies. Because of the serious nature of Accutane's side effects, make sure you have tried everything else possible before you use this medication.

◆ Differin. Differin is a topical prescription medication that's a Vitamin A derivative. It clears clogged pores but is gentle to the skin, and not as drying as Retin-A. Use as you would use Retin-A, being sure to always wear a high level of sun protection.

All of these products can ease or eliminate an acne flare-up. But none of them can kill off the p. acne for the rest of your life. Nothing can do that. The best thing you can do to eliminate future outbreaks is to make lifestyle changes.

Trigger Points

The first step in managing your lifestyle to prevent acne breakouts is to understand the circumstances that can trigger eruptions. Acne-type skin becomes more vulnerable to acne eruptions in certain conditions. Be sure you can either avoid these situations, or adapt to them to prevent eruptions.

◆ High stress levels. Flare-ups definitely occur with stress. Find ways to reduce stress through such activities as exercise, meditation, hobbies, and yoga. For more about stress-management choices, refer to Chapter 22.

◆ Hormonal changes. Many women experience acne eruptions in the week before their period starts. Teenagers often get acne eruptions as their adult reproductive hormones surge.

◆ Picking at eruptions. This can trigger a snowball effect. Picking at even one can trigger a whole rash of eruptions.

◆ Use of illegal drugs. Methamphetamine-type drugs, cocaine, and other strong stimulants can cause breakouts and keep them active. Absolutely stay away from these substances for the sake of your skin, your health, and, of course, your life.

◆ Legal stimulants. Substances such as coffee, caffeine, any kind of sodas, sugar, and regular tea can make a small breakout unmanageable. The stimulation increases the size, scope, and intensity of the outbreak.

◆ Smoking and alcoholic beverages. These make you more vulnerable to acne eruptions and can keep acne eruptions active. Stop smoking and drink alcoholic beverages infrequently, if at all.

◆ Certain work conditions. Working in a hot and humid environment, such as a restaurant kitchen, a factory, a dry cleaner, or a shirt laundry, can prompt acne eruptions.

◆ Certain types of clothing. A dental hygienist who regularly wears a face mask that rubs, a businessman who frequently wears a buttoned-up shirt with tie to the office, or any person who wears clothing that rubs and chafes can get acne in those areas.

◆ Vacation acne. If you vacation in the tropics or in warm and humid climates, you could get an acne eruption. You can avoid this by lightening up on moisturizer and doing more frequent exfoliation with a salicylic-BHA exfoliant.

◆ Eating a diet of junk food. Poor nutrition plays a huge role in being vulnerable to acne eruptions. Later in this chapter (see the section "Dietary Changes"), we tell you specifically what to eat to improve your diet as a way to manage acne eruptions.

◆ For no obvious reason. This is a tough one because sometimes, no matter what you do, you could have an eruption. However, chances are good that if you are doing everything right, any eruption will be minor and easily remedied.

Taking care to avoid these acne triggers is your first step in managing your skin. Later in this chapter (see the section "Making Lifestyle Changes"), you'll learn the specifics.

Acne Solutions

An excellent rule of thumb for any kind of skin condition is this: When it's on your skin, it started somewhere else in your body. By locating where the skin condition started, you can make corrections and see the resulting health on your skin.

Daily Care

In Chapter 3, you'll find a detailed description of how to care for acne-type skin. Here's a brief review:

◆ You need to clean twice a day and only twice a day. Blot excess oil with rice blotting papers as needed.

- Use a gel cleanser that contains salicylic acid.

- Use a toner that contains salicylic acid with a humectant. Apply with a spritz or a cotton pad.

- Use an oil-free moisturizer or one that contains tea tree oil. Apply lightly.

- Exfoliate two to three times a week with a chemical exfoliant containing BHA. Salicylic acid is BHA-beta hydroxy acid.

Be faithful to your daily routine. This will pay long-term dividends toward having clear skin.

Making Lifestyle Changes

Changing your lifestyle is your best acne remedy. Why? Because the results will be long-term and the changes you'll make are good for more than just your skin. Your overall mental and physical health will benefit as well.

Skin-spiration _____

Take care to keep bacteria from breeding on your skin care products. Wash cosmetic brushes and body buffers at least once a week. Only use a wash cloth or towel once before laundering. Never re-use face washing towelettes or wipes.

CAUTION   **Wrinkle Guard** _____

For acne-type skin, never go to sleep with a dirty face. Always cleanse, tone, and moisturize your face before bed. Sleeping with a dirty face encourages the p. acne bacteria to grow unchecked while you sleep.

Making lifestyle changes sounds easy, but it's often hard to do. Everyone has heard that they need to exercise for an hour every day, yet how many people actually exercise even three times a week? You know the answer—not many. Not even 20 percent of the population of the United States.

Most people with acne-type skin experience their first acne eruptions as teenagers. This is due to the upsurge of hormones in their bodies that begins with puberty. Perhaps the hardest time in life to make lifestyle changes is during the teenage years.

Yet, making those challenging and difficult changes can help avoid the tough psychological burden that comes with having active acne and the resultant lifelong scarring.

Teenagers want to fit in with their friends. They crave social acceptance and they want to hang out, eat junk food, drink sodas, and conform in every way possible. Therein lies the challenge. The lifestyle changes that are known to work preclude junk food and sodas (though not hanging out).

Even as an adult without the burden of peer-group acceptance, lifestyle changes can be challenging. They take time, planning, and plain old determination. Changing habits is difficult, but loving the results is easy.

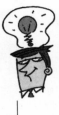

Skin-spiration

Teenagers who have acne-type skin need extra support to be able to make necessary lifestyle changes. If you are a parent, make sure that you stock up on foods teens should eat. Assist them with purchasing the skin care products that work best for their skin. Although at times it may not seem like they want it, they really do need your understanding and support.

Dietary Changes

What you put in your mouth can make all the difference in whether or not you have active or inactive acne. Foods that cause internal inflammation are the same foods that exaggerate acne breakouts.

Inflammation-causing foods are those that trigger a rapid rise in blood-sugar levels. When this happens, the pancreas gland excretes insulin. The insulin lowers the blood-sugar levels back to a healthy range, but in the process, the body experiences inflammation.

Wrinkle Guard

How you treat your skin today will make a big difference in how it looks years from now. Acne scarring lasts a lifetime. To avoid scarring, never pick at an eruption. In addition, eat the right foods and make the other lifestyle changes recommended in this chapter.

You can avoid inflammation by simply not eating the foods that cause this rapid rise in blood-sugar levels. Foods that are low on the glycemic index are the best for you to eat. High-glycemic foods are the worst for you to eat. We'll talk more about this whole process in Chapter 21.

Other inflammation-causing foods are any foods you are allergic to. Don't eat those foods. Eating them can trigger active acne.

Here are the foods to avoid:

◆ Pizza.

◆ Any kind of soda, both caffeinated and noncaffeinated, both diet and regular.

◆ Bread made with enriched or refined or white flour, including muffins, cookies, rice crackers, and crackers. You can eat whole grains and whole grain breads, providing that the ingredients don't contain enriched or white flour.

◆ Refined cereals and grains, such as breakfast cereals, both hot and cold. You can eat unrefined grains and cereals.

◆ Processed foods containing trans-fatty acids and partially hydrogenated vegetable oils.

◆ Dairy products, including cheese, milk, ice cream, and half and half.

- French fries and white potatoes.

- Coffee.

- Alcoholic beverages.

- Sugar and candy.

You may be wondering what's left to eat. Here are some suggestions:

- Meats, fish, poultry, seafood. Don't fry, but rather bake, grill, broil, or lightly sauté without breading.

- Vegetables. Bake, steam, broil, but don't fry. You can eat up to 10 servings a day. White potatoes don't count as a vegetable. You simply can't go wrong eating green vegetables.

- Fruit, with the exception of highly acidic fruits such as lemon, lime, grapefruits, and oranges.

- Nuts and seeds in their natural state—not highly salted. Avoid processed nut butters and instead use the natural types available at the health food store.

- Decaf tea and herbal teas.

- Eggs.

- Olive oil.

- Breads and cereals made from whole grains.

These foods aren't low carb, as the list contains plenty of good carbs, such as fruits and vegetables, but they definitely are low starch. Starches can cause inflammation.

The secret to making these foods work the best is to eat 5 to 10 servings of vegetables and/or fruits every day. They provide fiber and they give you plenty of antioxidants that nourish your skin.

What you can eat sparingly:

- Dark chocolate

- Decaf coffee

- Honey

- Butter

- Heavy cream

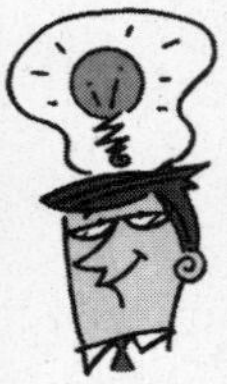

Skin-spiration

As you eat the foods that are good for acne-type skin, you may find that your clothes seem bigger. Yes, you're losing weight. These foods help people reach their ideal size and stay there almost effortlessly.

As you can see from the preceding lists, there's plenty of fabulous food you can eat. Even the fast-food restaurants are now offering foods with higher levels of nutrition, such as main-dish salads and hamburgers without the buns.

Can you get by with cheating a bit on your anti-eruption diet? Yes, a bit. Meaning that if you want a couple—say four or five French fries—once a week, you'll be fine. If you eat them every day, you won't like the results.

Nutritional Supplements

Nutritional supplements are vital for managing acne-type skin. Your skin will respond quickly when you start taking nutritional supplements that assure you're getting proper nutrition. Use the following supplements.

- Essential fatty acids, also known as EFAs. Found in salmon and sardines. Eat 2 to 5 servings of cold–water fish weekly to consume thee wonderful fats. Or you can supplement your diet with about 10 fish oil capsules or 2 tablespoons of a flaxseed-oil blend daily. Purchase at the health food store, grocery store, or discount chain.
- Acidophilus, the good bacteria that grows naturally in your intestinal tract. Depleted by the use of antibiotics and by stress. Also depleted by caffeinated beverages and alcoholic beverages. Helps prevent yeast overgrowth infections. Take a couple capsules a day, or as directed on package. You can also eat yogurt that contains active acidophilus cultures two to five times a week.
- Vitamin and mineral supplements. Gives you a balanced blend of B vitamins and minerals you need for basic health. Includes vitamins A, B5, B3, and B6, which specifically benefit acne-type skin. You can also add more of these four vitamins to your daily intake. These are best taken as a supplement.
- Zinc. Aids in the healing of tissue and helps prevent scarring. An important skin nutrient. Zinc is necessary for healthy oil-producing glands. It's found in egg yolks, fish, sardines, seafood, and pumpkin and sunflower seeds. As a supplement, don't take over 50 milligrams a day.
- Fiber. If you're eating five to ten servings of vegetables and fruits a day, you're already eating plenty of dietary fiber. You need about 25 to 35 grams a day. If you aren't, then use psyllium as a dietary supplement, available in bulk at health

food stores. Mix a spoonful in a glass of water and drink. Keeps elimination regular. Aids in detoxifying the body. Removes congestion from digestive tract.

◆ Digestive enzymes. If your stomach doesn't have adequate digestive enzymes, the undigested matter can try to come out through your skin. Take a general digestive enzyme tablet or capsule that includes digestive substances for proteins, fats, and carbohydrates. Take with each meal. Don't take between meals.

Take the above supplements daily and consistently. You might see a big improvement in a matter of days, but most likely in a matter of months. Natural healing works slowly at times, but it does work.

> **CAUTION**
>
> **Wrinkle Guard**
>
> It's only natural to have a bowel movement once or twice a day. Any less frequently than once a day can exacerbate an acne condition, because toxins and waste products aren't flowing normally from the body. Get regular and stay regular by eating plenty of fresh fruits and vegetables and taking fiber supplements as recommended here.

Exercise

Exercise is the easiest path to health and to healthy skin. It's easy because it's free, and you are guaranteed good results. Exercise increases your metabolism, brings healing oxygen to every cell, and makes you sweat. Sweating through the skin lets your pores normalize.

The thing about exercise that seems hard is actually setting aside the time and getting motivated to do it. Experts recommend that each of us exercise for an hour a day. To learn more about the benefits of exercise, refer to Chapter 24.

In short, here's what you need to do:

◆ Schedule your daily exercise session in your daily agenda. Keep the appointment with yourself.

◆ Exercise aerobically for at least three 20-minute sessions weekly.

◆ Do at least two strength training sessions a week of at least 30 minutes in duration. One hour is best.

◆ Stretch at least twice a week or 30 minutes each session.

Exercise makes your skin's oil flow. Because of this, your skin needs some special attention before and after you exercise. Pre-exercise, you can apply a moisturizer for oily skin that will absorb some of the oil flow. Post-exercise, wash your face if you can. If not, use pre-moisturized facial wipes made especially for oily skin. Then reapply your makeup. We don't recommend pre-moisturized facial wipes for regular daily cleansing, but they're great for special circumstances.

Beyond this listed minimum, you can always do more. Add in recreational exercise such as hiking, tennis, racquetball, or dancing.

Stress Makes Acne Worse

High stress levels can create inflammation that leads to acne eruptions. By now, you've probably experienced this. Perhaps during finals week at school, or the week before your wedding. It seems like acne eruptions happen when you need them the least. You're already too busy to deal with acne, and guess what? It shows up.

The high levels of the stress hormone cortisol and the resultant rise in insulin levels can cause eruptions and keep them coming. Your solution is to find ways to decompress every day. You can lower cortisol levels with activities such as yoga, meditation, exercise, and hobbies and crafts. These reduce stress. But sleeping on the sofa doesn't count, and neither does watching television. These in-activities don't lower cortisol levels. To learn more, refer to Chapter 22.

Professional Care for Acne

Skin care professionals can assist you in learning how to manage acne-type skin. You can work with both skin care technicians and dermatologists.

CAUTION

Wrinkle Guard

It's important to know that you can never cure acne-type skin. You'll always have it. While medication or a facial can help heal a current eruption, it can't cure your skin. Only by changing your eating habits and other lifestyle factors can you successfully manage acne-type skin for life.

Skin care technicians usually work at salons or spas. They're licensed by the state and have extensive training in skin and skin care. A skin care technician can give you a facial, which includes cleaning out your pores and removing whiteheads and blackheads. They can do this safely without causing disruption to your skin and they work with sterilized tools. Your facial can include masks and peels that detoxify your skin.

A skin care technician can give you personalized instruction in how to care for your skin, as he or she will learn exactly how your skin behaves and understand how to manage your skin.

A dermatologist is a doctor who specializes in skin conditions. If you have active acne, you need to see a dermatologist. He or she can prescribe an antibiotic or Retin-A. In the most severe cases, he or she may recommend the medication Accutane.

If you have a large acne cyst or pustule, the dermatologist can inject the spot with cortisone, which reduces inflammation. Some dermatologists will cut out a cyst with a scalpel as a last resort and only after the cyst has been repeatedly inflamed. Removing a cyst creates a scar that doesn't go away.

Psychologically Speaking

Active acne takes its toll on a person's self-esteem and self-confidence. It looks bad. It's embarrassing. It can mean the difference between being hired and being rejected. It can be the difference between being socially accepted by one's peers or being an outcast. It's easy to say that beauty is only skin deep, but the truth is that it's hard to live with active acne and with acne scars.

If active acne is damaging your psyche, schedule a trip to a psychiatrist or psychologist to learn how to manage your attitude and sense of self-worth. It will be a good investment in your future.

Next, take action. Taking action puts depression and self-doubt at bay as you take positive steps to remedying the situation. Follow the steps outlined in this chapter as a start. Then get on with living a full and wonderful life. You can do it!

Acne-Scarring Solutions

For every legitimate way to reduce acne scarring, there are hundreds of expensive scams. A person who has acne scarring is especially vulnerable to scams that promise to completely eliminate unsightly and embarrassing scars. Fortunately, most skin discolorations due to acne fade with time and don't need surgical treatments. To hasten their fading, you can use hydroquinone or a skin-lightening formulation with licorice.

Light scarring often responds well to retinol, available over the counter and to topical Vitamin A derivatives, the prescription medications Retin-A and Renova.

In actuality, some scars can be removed and some can't. Ask a dermatologist for the best approach to removing or minimizing acne scars.

- ◆ Keloid scars are caused by increased tissue formation. You can be genetically predisposed to keloid formation. When a pimple or other insult doesn't heal properly, the body produces excess collagen which forms into fibrous red-brown lumps. They're most common in people of color, but anyone can have the genetic programming that forms keloids. Correction can be tricky. Cutting them out usually creates another keloid. Cortisone injections may flatten them and reduce redness. These types of acne scars are caused by tissue loss.

◆ Dell scars are shallow depressions with smooth edges and can make your skin look rippled or wavy. Ragged-edged scars are shallow depressions with uneven or ragged edges. Microdermabrasion can soften these. Laser resurfacing and Thermage can also help. Injections with Restylane and other fillers can work. Restylane is a temporary solution and lasts about six months to a year. Make sure you aren't allergic to any permanent fillers because if you are, they have to be cut out, making yet another scar.

◆ Ice-pick scars are small, deep holes with ragged edges. Over time, they can become depressed fibrotic scars with larger, deep holes and ragged edges. Removal of these types of scars requires surgery to either sew them up or to fill the holes with skin tissue removed from another place on the body, usually from behind the ears.

◆ Sinus tracts are spaghetti-like tunnels under the skin that connect sebaceous glands. Surgery to correct these scars usually leads to more scarring and can even promote new acne cyst formation.

◆ Follicular macular atrophy resembles whiteheads and is usually found on the back and chest. Acne scars on the body are more difficult to remedy than those on the face. Some people have had success with pulse-dye laser to relieve redness. Lightening products such as hydroquinone can lighten dark spots. Use fillers, such as Restylane to fill depressions on the face.

Ask your dermatologist or doctor what you can realistically expect to remove acne scars. It may not be realistic to expect all acne scars to totally disappear, but you may find that some scars can be softened and that some can be erased. If you choose to have either of these procedures done, be sure to check practitioners' references and actually talk with acne clients and find out if they're happy with the results. Seek out a doctor who has done many scar removal procedures and who has excellent references. Avoid anyone who promises you a miracle.

Beware of anyone who tells you they have a special system that removes acne scarring. Most likely you're being conned. Some scams involve using 70 percent glycolic acid on the skin or electrical wave machines. If you feel too much pressure to buy, the hard sell is a good indication that you should go home fast.

Before you have any scar removal work done, make sure that you are taking good daily care of your skin, that you are exfoliating regularly, and that you've made the lifestyle changes recommended in this chapter. Give your skin time to normalize and find out how much healing it can do on its own. Then you can determine if you can comfortably live with your skin exactly the way it is.

If you still decide you want to have some scars removed, check out dermabrasion, microdermabrasion, and laser resurfacing. Ask your dermatologist or skin care technician for references. Be aware that health insurance seldom pays for this form of cosmetic surgery.

You may also want to learn how to apply medical-type makeup to cover up scars. When applied well, today's formulations can make your skin look radiant and much smoother.

The Least You Need to Know

- Acne is a skin condition that's most susceptible to the p. acne bacteria that grows on and under the surface of the skin.

- There are six grades of acne, ranging from inactive to active with cysts, pustules, papules, blackheads, and whiteheads.

- Never pick at an acne eruption because you can create dozens more from one squeeze.

- Making changes in diet, exercise, stress levels, and nutritional supplementation can calm acne and reduce eruptions.

- Go to the dermatologist if you have active acne eruptions.

Chapter 12

Congestion, Breakouts, and Irritation

In This Chapter

- Identifying breakouts, congestion, and irritation
- Determining the root causes
- Skin care for breakouts and congestion
- Aids for prevention

The occasional breakout can happen to anyone—regardless of skin type. A pimple or two doesn't mean you technically have acne, it simply means your skin has a breakout. Don't panic. If you do the right things as soon as you spot a blemish, it can vanish within days.

Congested skin seems dull, sluggish, and rough to the touch. Your skin is no longer dewy, moist, and plump. You could have blackheads or whiteheads. The skin feels bumpy, and milia could be present. Your skin can seem irritated with a rash. Like a breakout, congested skin is a temporary condition that can be remedied quickly.

In this chapter, we show you how to clear up congestion and breakouts, plus what lifestyle changes you can make to prevent them.

Breaking Out

Everyone gets skin breakouts or congested skin from time to time, no matter what their skin type. Even normal-type skin can break out and become congested. Breakouts can be caused by shifting hormonal levels or a visit to a much more humid climate. You can also get breakouts and congestion from airplane travel and high stress levels.

Men, if you have breakouts, check to make sure you have a new blade in your razor and that your shirt collar isn't rubbing on your neck. If you wear starched shirts and you have a rash on your neck, try unstarched shirts for a couple of weeks and see if the breakout goes away. Also, be sure you aren't using deodorant soap to wash you face. It's a guaranteed irritant.

> **⚠ CAUTION**
>
> ### Wrinkle Guard
>
> Don't stop taking your prescription medications to improve the appearance of your skin. This could be dangerous to your health. Instead, consult with your doctor and your pharmacist to determine if your medication can cause congested skin. If so, ask if there is a substitute that could be gentler.

Using illegal drugs and certain prescription medications can give you breakouts or congestion, as can alcoholic beverages. Your body uses up valuable B vitamins as well as other vitamins and minerals to deal with these substances. Those nutrients then aren't available for healthy skin functioning. The liver is overtaxed in detoxifying from these substances and has less availability to detoxify normal skin wastes. Avoid habits such as these that can trigger breakouts.

Breakouts are only temporary conditions. You can break out of breaking out by fixing what's wrong, by using careful skin management, and, of course, by making lifestyle changes.

What's in a Pimple

A pimple starts forming when a pore gets closed off, often as the result of built up dead skin cells, waste products, and sebum. Sebum gets trapped inside the pore. The body's immune system sends in white blood cells as protection, which is good. But those white blood cells also create inflammation.

As a pimple becomes inflamed, bacteria rush to the pimple to feast on the inflammation. It's not a pretty picture, but this is what is happening in your skin. The bacteria that could be growing include p. acne, staphylococcus, streptococcus, or herpes. You could also have a yeast infection.

These are serious bacteria, so you absolutely don't want to pick at your skin and perhaps cause them to spread into your bloodstream. The areas most likely to spread bacteria to the blood stream are around your nose and upper lip because these are close to the mucous membranes.

Skin-spiration

Here's a simple home remedy for healing a pimple. Take a regular uncoated aspirin. Dip in water, then rub the pimple with the aspirin. Leave on overnight and the next morning, your pimple may be totally gone. If not, repeat until pimple is cleared. Or you can crush an aspirin and mix with a very small amount of water to make a paste, then apply to skin. The salicylic acid in the aspirin exfoliates the dead skin cells above the pimple and kills the bacteria.

If your pimple or breakout looks serious or unusual, go directly to the phone and set an appointment with a dermatologist for that day or the next. Don't delay and don't wait for the breakout to get better. You may require medical care.

Congested Skin

The life span of a skin cell is 28 days in younger people and up to 40 days in older people. In that time span, a skin cell is formed, does its work, dies off, and is then replaced by another skin cell. Healthy skin naturally sheds the dead skin and reveals fresh new skin cells.

This process only works partway in congested skin. The skin cells die naturally and are replaced, but the dead skin cells aren't sloughed off. They build up on the surface of the skin.

As a result, pores get clogged up and the skin becomes congested. The natural sebum and oils on the skin can't get out of the pores, so they build up and, voilà, you guessed it, the buildup becomes whiteheads and blackheads.

Body of Knowledge

Congestion can occur on any body area. When congestion occurs on the upper arms, shoulders, buttocks, and thighs, the condition is called keratosis pilaris and is characterized by whiteheads—hard, clogged pores that form bumps. This may be an inherited condition. Exfoliating with glycolic or lactic acid works to clear them. Also, these bumps can be caused by poor digestion, in which waste products are excreted through the pores. Try taking a digestive enzyme supplement that includes hydrochloric betaine with each meal, and within a couple of weeks the bumps could disappear.

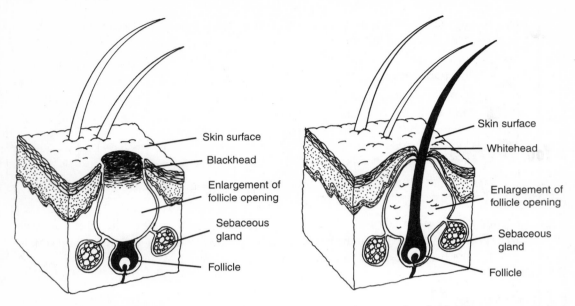

A diagram of a blackhead.   *A diagram of a whitehead.*

Congestion is usually temporary and can be caused by many different health and lifestyle situations. Some include hormonal imbalances, such as a thyroid imbalance, sickness, using the wrong cosmetics, smoking, pollution, and friction from clothing. An example of friction is the chafing that can occur when frequently wearing a face-mask, as dental hygienists do.

Congestion occurs in all skin types. Most of the time, congestion is only temporary and can be corrected by using the suggestions in this chapter. But if you smoke, you can have continual congestion, reflected in dull and lifeless skin.

Clarifying Words

Milia are small, whitish, hard, pearl-like bumps in the skin due to retention of sebum. Another name for milia is white-heads.

When you touch congested skin, it's somewhat rough with dead skin cells, tiny whiteheads (called *milia*), and blackheads. It can make you feel like you just want to scrub your face until it comes clean. Don't do this, as there are much more elegant and effective solutions.

Correcting the Condition

You need to take positive action quickly to remedy breakouts, congestion, or irritation. Because the condition is temporary, be positive. Yes, it's possible that breakouts or congestion will recur in the future, but if and when this happens, you'll know exactly what to do and what not to do.

Your First Step

The first step in solving breakouts, irritations, and congestion is to determine what's causing the condition. Review any changes you've made in the past month or so. Such changes might include the following:

- Illness.
- Travel.
- Vacations.
- Skipping your daily skin ritual.
- New laundry detergent.
- Laundry detergent with bleaches and fragrances.
- New perfume or aftershave.
- Smoking, drug usage.
- Lack of sleep.
- Air fresheners, candles, incense.
- Change of diet.
- Dehydration, or not drinking enough pure water.
- Aromatherapy.
- New skin care products.
- Yeast infections that can cause rashes, flaking, and pimples.
- Eating a high-starch or high-sugar diet.
- Change in stress levels.
- Allergic reactions to new carpet, furniture, or floor coverings.
- Allergic reactions to new bedding, pillows.

◆ Constipation, diarrhea, indigestion.

◆ Some over-the-counter medications, such as cortisone cream, benzoyl peroxide, chemical sunscreens, Neosporin, Icy-Hot. But you can react to virtually any topical over-the-counter medication, as well as to any that you take orally.

◆ Muscle aches due to build up of lactic acid following strength-training exercise. Lactic acid buildup can cause your body to get overly acidic. The overly acidic condition causes congestion and breakouts.

Go through this list and identify what has changed in your life or habits. You're not limited to what's in this list. Try to identify any changes in your routine or added stresses that you've recently experienced.

Skin-spiration

Sue was really into natural health and healing. A friend suggested she sip on a daily tonic of fresh-squeezed lemon, lime, and orange juice sweetened with maple syrup and spiced with one-half teaspoon cayenne. Within three days, Sue had blemishes and very tender skin. The potion may have been healthy for others, but Sue's only results were breakouts and congestion. By discontinuing her daily tonic, her skin healed. Even things that seem to be good for you can cause breakouts and congestion.

When you identify what's causing congestion or breakouts, make positive changes immediately. Eliminate things that are affecting you negatively, and if you've made positive changes in your lifestyle that are showing up on your skin, be extra diligent about your skin care routine. Remember, breakouts and congestion are *temporary*.

Some life conditions can't be changed easily, and some you don't want to change:

◆ Air pollution or temperature inversion in your city

◆ New working condition or new job

◆ Move to new home or new city

◆ Pregnancy or hormonal changes

◆ Prescription medications

◆ New pet, such as a cat or dog

◆ Marriage, divorce, new companion

◆ Change of seasons

With these situations, you may need to adapt. For example, if you know that you get breakouts or congestion before your menstrual periods start, plan for it. Take impeccable daily care of your skin and exfoliate more frequently. Lighten up on foods and beverages that can cause congestion at those times. Rest more. Exercise more. You may need to change air filters in your home more frequently. And make sure to change the filters on your water softeners and water purifiers frequently. Take positive action to reduce stress and your skin will look better in no time. See Part 5 for lifestyle and diet suggestions to reduce congestion, irritations, and breakouts.

The Picking Problem

It's so tempting to pick at skin breakouts, whiteheads, and blackheads. Yes, you want them out of your skin. All we can say is: Don't do it! Your picking could result in scarring and even more breakouts. Refer to Chapter 11 for details.

If you are desperate to have your skin cleaned out, schedule a facial with a licensed skin care technician. He or she knows exactly how to do extractions that help heal your skin. A skin technician always uses sterilized tools and wears protective gloves to protect your face from any germs and bacteria that could be on his or her hands.

In addition to whitehead, blackhead, and pimple extraction, a facial includes exfoliation and a detoxifying mask. You'll leave with skin that feels fresh, clean, and radiant.

An at-home solution is to zap your zit with a drop of salicylic acid. It may be all you need to clean out the pimple. Also, when you aren't going out, apply a small amount of clay mask just to the zit. It dries it up and speeds recovery.

Otherwise, use concealer as you take steps to correct your skin condition. Just be sure to wash it off every evening before bed.

CAUTION

Wrinkle Guard

Be sure you don't exfoliate too frequently. You could disrupt the acid mantle of the skin and invite infections and inflammation. Too frequently depends on your skin and its needs. If you usually exfoliate three times a week, you could increase that to four times the week before your menstrual cycle. Be sure not to overdo it.

Skin-spiration

If you have a really bad breakout—such as a stubborn bright red pimple—you can visit the dermatologist for an injection of cortisone directly into the pimple. The cortisone reduces the inflammation. We don't recommend you do this frequently, but if you're on your way to the altar or a terrifically big life-changing event, by all means, go to the dermatologist.

The Healing Step

Your skin needs a good round of regular, and possibly even more frequent, exfoliation for a couple of days, perhaps even for a week or two. You need to get those dead skin cells off the surface of your skin and allow the newer, fresher skin cells to glow.

You can rotate using several different kinds of exfoliators. You might use a salicylic acid one day, then switch to an enzyme exfoliant two days later. Two days after that, use a gentle scrub with polyurethane beads or corn meal. If your skin starts looking red, ease up and give it time to calm down and heal. More exfoliation will cause further irritation and inflammation, and, as you can guess, more problems.

At the Same Time

Be sure you continue to faithfully cleanse, tone, and moisturize each morning and evening. If you aren't satisfied with the outcome, it may be time to change skin care products. They may not meet your skin's needs any longer. This can happen when you change activity level, with health-related changes, with pregnancy, or even as you age. Moving to a city with more or less humidity can even change your skin's needs.

If you've been faithful to your skin care regimen before and during the breakout or congestion, and you can't identify the cause of your skin condition, it may be time to modify your skin care products.

> **CAUTION**
> **Wrinkle Guard**
>
> Even though you may want to clear up a breakout or congestion quickly, and feel like you should cleanse, tone, and moisturize more than twice a day, don't. This causes even more irritation and inflammation, plus dryness. You might actually make your skin problems worse. Be gentle. In this case, more isn't necessarily better.

First of all, check with your sales consultant and ask him or her to look at your face. You may need a different product formulation, or you may even need to change skin care lines. Go slowly here. When your skin is in a vulnerable situation, you may not want to radically change your skin products, because the change might stress your skin further. On the other hand, it may be necessary to clear up new problems. Get advice. If you change to new products and you get a bad reaction, return the products and start over. If the congestion, irritation, and breakouts continue, set up a consultation with a skin care specialist or a dermatologist.

Add-On Solutions

In addition to all the actions in this chapter, you can add in some extra activities that will help your skin stay healthy.

◆ Spend a whole day relaxing. Read a novel. Take walks. Coddle yourself and reduce your stress levels. In other words, take a vacation day and stay at home.

◆ Sweat. Get out and exercise until you break a sweat and keep on moving. Go to the sauna or steam room. Take a Bikram yoga class where the room temperature is kept hot on purpose. Be sure to cleanse your face after strenuous exercise.

◆ Add lots of fiber to your diet to help excrete toxins from your body. A spoonful of psyllium husks, a non-calorie bulk fiber supplement available at the health food store, in a glass of water works great and is healthy for you. You can mix this up and take it before bed or any other time of the day. Follow with a glass of water.

◆ Stretch your body. Stretching feels great and helps your body detoxify. You can choose from regular yoga classes, Pilates classes, or simply stretch out every evening at home.

◆ Drink at least 64 ounces of purified water daily. Use an electrolyte supplement such as Emergen-C to help you stay hydrated.

◆ Change stressful situations that you can. This could mean ending a relationship that doesn't work or apologizing after a fight even if you feel you were in the right,

> **CAUTION** **Wrinkle Guard**
>
> If you have a really odd or abnormal skin eruption or lesion, go immediately to the dermatologist. You need a professional consultation as soon as possible.

These add-on solutions are meant to be fun—so relax. When you reduce your overall stress levels and take better care of yourself physically and emotionally, your skin will remain calm and clear. Your efforts will end the crisis soon.

Calming Cold Sores

Cold sores are a different type of breakout. The sore, usually on the lip or mouth area, is caused by herpes simplex type 1 virus. The virus can remain dormant in your body for years, and suddenly erupt, often with the onset of heavy-duty stress or exposure to ultraviolet light. Other known triggers are waxing, chemical peels, laser treatments, and Retin-A.

When you feel the tingling sensation that first comes with a herpes eruption, the following are options:

◆ Use a prescription medication such as Zovirax, Valtrex, or Famvir to forestall a full eruption.

◆ Take the amino acid, L-lysine, and some extra B vitamins. Some people swear by these natural remedies for thwarting an eruption.

◆ Have a skin care specialist use a high-frequency light machine to aid in healing the sore.

The Least You Need to Know

◆ Breakouts and congestion are conditions that occur in all skin types.

◆ Identify the root causes of breakouts and congestion so you can manage or avoid them.

◆ Consult with a dermatologist for serious breakouts.

◆ Never pick at a pimple, blackhead, or whitehead.

Rosacea

In This Chapter

- ◆ Recognizing rosacea
- ◆ Managing rosacea flare-ups
- ◆ Consulting with a dermatologist
- ◆ Making lifestyle changes

There are many misconceptions about rosacea, including the most basic concern: what it is. Some people—even some skin care specialists—think of it as acne for grownups. Not true. In fact, if you treat rosacea as you would treat acne, most likely your skin condition will get worse.

W. C. Fields, the comedian and actor, had rosacea. He played up his enlarged red nose as a sign of living a hard-drinking life. Certainly, alcohol can exacerbate the condition of rosacea, but the use of alcoholic beverages doesn't actually cause rosacea. But it sure can cause flare-ups.

In this chapter, you'll learn the current research about rosacea and the most effective treatment methods. Experts aren't sure what causes rosacea and some now think that it could be several different skin conditions. At present, no one knows how to cure it, but new treatments combined with gentle care and lifestyle changes can put the condition into remission indefinitely.

The Skin Disorder of Rosacea

Rosacea is an inflammatory blood vessel and capillary disorder that occurs mostly in adults. It's most common in people of Celtic and Scandinavian descent. Rosacea appears on the face, and can also appear on the neck, chest, scalp, or ears. Most often, the first signs of rosacea are frequent flushing or blushing that lasts longer than normal. The condition can progress to bumps, pimples, and visible blood vessels that lie under the surface of the skin.

Rosacea is characterized by flare-ups and remissions. Flare-ups can be reduced and minimized by making lifestyle changes.

Symptoms of rosacea include the following:

◆ Flushing skin

◆ Persistent redness and inflammation

◆ Unexplained bumps and pimples that aren't from acne, congestion, or normal breakouts

◆ Visible blood vessels or spider veins

◆ Eye irritation

◆ Burning or stinging skin

◆ Rough facial skin that appears very dry

◆ Raised red patches, also known as plaques

◆ Skin thickening on the nose or cheeks

◆ Facial swelling

CAUTION

Wrinkle Guard

If someone other than a dermatologist suggests your skin condition is rosacea, be wary. Instead, you may have breakouts, congestion, sunburn, windburn, or acne. Or you could simply be using the wrong skin care product. All of these conditions can look similar to rosacea. If you are concerned, visit a dermatologist and get a professional opinion.

If you have persistent unexplained redness, stinging, or burning in your skin, visit a dermatologist right away. Early diagnosis and treatment can arrest the development of rosacea and prevent it from reaching the more acute stages.

The Causes of Rosacea

Medical and skin care experts aren't in agreement about what rosacea is. Some think that what is known as rosacea could actually be one of three separate skin disorders. Here are the most probable causes:

◆ The human demodex mite. About 97 percent of all people host the mite in their skin, but in some people the mite grows out of control under the skin of the face. No one is certain why the demodex mite grows out of control in some people causing rosacea and not in others, but genetics seems to play a role. Many people who have rosacea caused by the demodex mite are experiencing great results by using new products that actually kill the mites. These products are formulated with sea buckthorn berry essential oil, tea tree oil, or sea whip. Sea whip is a marine animal.

◆ A gastro-intestinal organism that triggers an autoimmune disorder. Research studies haven't yet proven this theory or shown how to heal it.

◆ P. acne bacteria. Unfortunately, skin treatments for p. acne don't work well for rosacea and, in fact, seem to aggravate it for most people. However, some people can use mild acne products to reduce redness and breakouts.

If you suspect that you have rosacea, you may need to try several approaches before you find the one that works for you. Rosacea is tricky to care for, so you may want to get several opinions and treatment recommendations.

Stages of Rosacea

Rosacea is a progressive condition. A person may progress through all four stages, or the condition can remain at any one stage.

Stage One: Skin flushes or blushes. Your skin is persistently red, and may have visible blood vessels. At first, your symptoms could be as simple as your face getting really red from drinking alcohol, eating spicy hot foods, using a sauna, or following exposure to the sun's ultraviolet radiation. Your face swells a little, but eventually your skin returns to normal. Other activities that can prompt Stage One are hot yoga, high-level aerobic exertion, or anything that heats up the body, such as spending time in a hot tub, steam room, or taking a hot bath.

Stage Two: The capillaries stay red and spider veins form. Your nose and cheeks stay red, or flushed, most of the time. Bumps or pimples may appear from time to time. Your skin is not painful, but the condition is annoying. Many people with rosacea stay at this stage indefinitely.

Stage Three: The face is very red and has become painful to the touch. It could hurt to smile. The blood vessels have lost their elasticity. Blood can pool just under the skin causing the appearance of bruising. Because there's damage to blood vessels, the lymph system becomes less effective at carrying away toxins. The skin gets thicker, resulting in enlargement of some areas of the face, most often the cheeks or nose. W. C. Fields was an example of a person with Stage Three rosacea.

Clarifying Words

Edema is an abnormal swelling of the fluid in the tissues. A **stye** is an inflammation of one of the sebaceous glands of the eyelid.

Stage Four: Full-blown rosacea. The last stage is quite serious. Your eyes become dry with tearing and burning, and may swell shut with *edema*. *Styes* in the eyes can lead to potential vision loss. The skin is always inflamed, and is crusty and scaly, with persistent pain.

Although a sure cure for rosacea hasn't been found, you can use some of the newest treatment products as well as stop the progression of rosacea by making lifestyle changes. We'll explore this further as we continue.

Who's Susceptible to Rosacea

Virtually anyone can have rosacea, but some groups of people are far more susceptible to it.

◆ Rosacea usually shows up in adults and less frequently in teenagers and children.

◆ People with sensitive skin types are more likely to have rosacea.

◆ Caucasians with fair hair and skin are more likely to get rosacea, leading some experts to think that a person could be genetically predisposed to rosacea.

◆ Menopausal women are more likely to have rosacea, and it's thought to be provoked by hot flashes that result from low estrogen levels.

◆ Both men and women can have rosacea. Men usually have rosacea most noticeably on the nose, which can become enlarged. Women with rosacea usually notice it first on the nose, but then it spreads to the cheeks.

This list gives you a sense of the people who are most likely to develop rosacea; however, it can develop in anyone, and it's to everyone's benefit to know how to manage it and keep rosacea in remission should it occur in the future.

Regular Skin Care for Rosacea

Rosacea seems like a mysterious condition, especially if you have it. The very treatments that a person would normally use for breakouts or acne won't work for rosacea. In fact, they can aggravate the condition and make it worse. Prior to home treatment, visit a dermatologist to confirm that you have rosacea. You could possibly have another skin condition that requires very different treatment.

Investigate new treatments for rosacea that include products formulated with the ingredients of sea buckthorn berry essential oil, sea whip, or tea tree oil. All of these ingredients are widely available and you don't need a prescription to use them. As with all products that touch your skin, start first with a patch test for three days before applying to your entire face.

The most important factor in your daily skin care routine is to be gentle with your skin. You still need to cleanse, tone, and moisturize twice a day, but use a gentle lotion cleanser and avoid the stronger gel cleansers. Don't use salicylic acid cleaners. Use a gentle toner with humectants that don't contain alcohol. Use a gentle moisturizer without fragrances that can irritate your skin.

> **Skin-spiration**
>
> If your skin care technician or dermatologist isn't familiar with the demodex mite, you may want to consult with someone who is. You can also use the Internet to research treatments and products.

For exfoliators, avoid chemical exfoliants that contain glycolic acid, though lactic acid is gentle enough for your skin. Avoid exfoliants that are too stimulating for your skin. Don't use scrubs or enzymes. Instead, exfoliate using a soothing oatmeal mask or any other nondrying mask with anti-inflammatory ingredients like aloe, raspberry, or *allantion*.

> **Clarifying Words**
>
> **Allantion** is a derivative of uric acid that is soothing and calming to the skin. It's found in roots, bark, and grains, and is used in skin products for healing.

If any of your skin care products are irritating or cause inflammation, stop using them and switch to a product that's gentler for your skin. Here's a list of products and ingredients that can make rosacea worse:

- Ultraviolet light (always wear a sunscreen)
- Benzocaine
- Benzoyl peroxide
- Corticosteroids (such as cortisone cream)
- Hydrogen peroxide
- Hydroquinone
- Methosalicylate
- Some chemical sunscreens (instead use sun blocks such as zinc oxide and titanium dioxide—mineral powder makeups and sun blocks are cooling and work well for persons with rosacea)

- ◆ Resourcinol

- ◆ Retin A, Accutane, Renova, Differin, and all retinoids

- ◆ Salicylic acid

- ◆ Antibacterial soaps

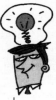

Skin-spiration _____

Some skin care products are formulated to meet the needs of rosacea. Ask your dermatologist or a skin care technician for product recommendations. Be sure to ask about using products with sea buckthorn berry and sea whip. You can also do a search online for rosacea skin care products. If you purchase, make sure you can return them if you find them irritating or if they aren't effective for you.

When trying out any new products for the condition of rosacea, be sure to go slow. Do a patch test for several days to make sure that your skin won't react negatively to the product.

Use a nonirritating foundation and concealer. You may also want to use a heavier cover-up concealer when you have a flare-up. Here are some ingredients used in cosmetics that may trigger rosacea flare-ups:

- ◆ Alpha hydroxyl acids

- ◆ Arachadonic acid

- ◆ Ascorbic acid

- ◆ DMAE

- ◆ Some essential oils

- ◆ Formaldehyde

- ◆ Fruit enzymes

- ◆ Niacin

- ◆ Peanut and sesame oil

- ◆ Propylene glycol

- ◆ Sulfur

- ◆ Sodium lauryl or sodium laureth sulfate

Skin-spiration _____

Stress is a significant culprit in rosacea flare-ups. If you are prone to such stress-induced behaviors as panic attacks, mania, or anxiety attacks, take positive actions to learn how to manage these stress-provoked behaviors. You may want to learn behavior modification techniques or consult with a psychiatrist to learn new and calming coping strategies.

Use the same strategy with cosmetics that you do with skin care products. Do a skin patch test for at least three days to determine how your skin reacts to the product. If you have a flare up at the test spot, don't use the product. You could also determine that other substances not listed here trigger flare-ups for you.

If you have pimples and bumps associated with rosacea, never disturb them. Picking can make your skin condition worse and could be so irritating that you provoke your condition to progress to the next stage of severity. Instead, continue with your regular skin care routine.

> **CAUTION**
>
> **Wrinkle Guard**
>
> When you have pimples, pustules, or papules from rosacea, don't use salicylic acid to zap them. You could make things worse. Instead, use a clay mask to deep clean your skin.

Medical Treatments

Your dermatologist can prescribe medications to help reduce the symptoms of rosacea. These include cortisone to reduce swelling and inflammation and antibiotics to kill off bacteria in the pimples, pustules, and papules. If your rosacea is painful, ask which pain relievers your dermatologist recommends.

Medications to avoid are topical steroids. They may help reduce symptoms initially but can create severe problems over time. Also avoid acne treatments. Rosacea used to be called "acne rosacea" and was treated the same as acne. Today, we know that rosacea is a very different condition than acne and must be treated differently. Benzoyl peroxide, a common ingredient in acne preparations, can make rosacea symptoms worse.

For more advanced stages of rosacea, treatments with lasers or other medical devices like intense pulsed light may be beneficial. These treatments can remove visible blood vessels, reduce redness, and correct disfigurement of the nose.

If your eyes are affected by rosacea, ask your dermatologist for treatment. He or she may prescribe oral antibiotics or other medications.

Avoiding Flare-Ups

First and foremost, stay away from the activities that aggravate rosacea and cause flare-ups. These include doing anything that raises body temperature.

◆ Avoid hot showers, the sauna, hot tubs, and hot baths. Avoid physical exertion that elevates body temperature. Yes, do exercise, but do more gentle aerobics.

- ◆ Avoid overexertion as it can cause your body temperature to rise too much.

- ◆ Avoid sun exposure and avoid exposure to winds, especially cold winds. These can trigger flare-ups.

- ◆ Avoid foods and substances that aggravate rosacea. These include alcoholic beverages and smoking.

- ◆ Avoid caffeine in coffee and tea, and also in sodas and diet sodas.

- ◆ Avoid eating highly spicy foods, such as Mexican or Thai cuisines.

- ◆ Avoid using hot pepper, such as cayenne, when cooking. Sometimes citric fruits, such as lemons, limes, grapefruit, and oranges can aggravate rosacea.

- ◆ Avoid hot beverages, and instead drink at least eight glasses of purified water every day. The water moves toxins and waste products from the body, keeps bowel movements regular, and transports nutrients throughout your body.

- ◆ Avoid household products that contain harsh detergents, and keep fragrances like perfume and cologne away from your skin.

- ◆ Avoid using a face or body towel more than once. Make sure you launder after each use.

Men may want to use an electric shaver rather than a razor for shaving. Maintain or adopt healthy eating patterns. Eat 5 to 10 servings of vegetables and fruits daily. Take 2 tablespoons of essential fatty acids daily. Eat cold-water fish like salmon or sardines two or three times a week. Stay away from the foods that cause inflammation, such as breads, pasta, wheat, rice, cookies, muffins, and bagels. Avoiding dairy products, sugar, and chocolate may also help avoid flare-ups.

Keep a food and activity journal to track what causes rosacea flare-ups for you. Ultimately, only you can know what works and doesn't work for you and the health of your skin.

At the Salon

A good skin care specialist won't do extractions on rosacea. However, skin care specialists can do lymphatic drainage that assists in removing toxins and waste products from the skin. This feels great and is very soothing, which is just what your skin and your psyche need.

Ask the technician to teach you how to do manual lymphatic drainage for yourself. Remember to always use a light touch. This can help your skin feel and look better.

A skin care technician can also give you a gentle facial and apply a soothing and cooling mask to your skin. Other soothing spa treatments include a cold-marble stone treatment or lymphatic massage. A cold-marble stone treatment is cooling to the skin. It reduces inflammation, stops the burn of rosacea, and calms the skin. Lymphatic massage gently stimulates the lymph fluid to remove toxins from the surface of the skin. Light pressure is applied to lymph nodes around the neck, head, and face.

Your dermatologist may recommend laser treatments to dissolve spider veins and broken capillaries under the skin. This works very well for some people, but not for everyone.

The Least You Need to Know

- ◆ Rosacea is a skin condition with no known cause and no known cure.

- ◆ A person can manage rosacea and keep it in remission though daily cleansing and making lifestyle changes.

- ◆ Rosacea can be mistaken for acne, but rosacea needs to be treated very differently.

- ◆ See a dermatologist if you suspect you have rosacea.

Dehydrated Skin

In This Chapter

- Identifying dehydration
- Finding the root causes
- Making lifestyle changes
- Special moisturizing treatments

Today, millions of people lay claim to having dry skin. And there are certainly thousands of skin care products formulated and marketed especially for dry skin. Yet, as a genetic skin type, dry skin by itself doesn't exist. What *does* exist is the skin condition of dehydrated skin. If you are an oil-dry skin type, you may or may not be dehydrated.

Anyone with any skin type can have dehydrated skin. Your skin feels dry and tight. When you smile, it seems like your face cracks. Your skin tone has changed from bright and clear to ashen and dull. It's likely that your skin is dehydrated.

Unfortunately, none of the dry-skin moisturizers and treatments alone can correct dehydrated skin. They can only help. Correcting dehydrated skin requires you to change your environment and make lifestyle changes.

Only a Temporary Condition

Perhaps your skin has gotten drier as you have gotten older. Or maybe it seems like no amount of moisturizer makes a difference. Your face still feels dry.

Dehydrated skin is dry to the touch. It may itch. You might have flaky patches and rough spots, and you might see blotchy patches when you look in the mirror. Your skin tone lacks vibrancy and radiance.

If your skin remains dehydrated for too long, *keratinization* can occur. The dead skin cells build up on the surface of your skin until they coat it, making it nearly impossible for moisturizer to reach your skin. Your skin gets more dehydrated. With keratinization come congestion and breakouts. Your skin is crying out for moisture.

The good news is that dehydration is only a temporary condition, no matter what your age. Your skin can quickly rehydrate and can start to function as healthy skin once again.

> **Clarifying Words**
>
> **Keratinization** is the development of a rough quality in skin tissue. Keratin is a protein cell in skin tissue. Keratin is made soluble with AHAs and BHAs, and can be broken down by enzyme exfoliants.

> **Wrinkle Guard**
>
> Forget about searching through the stores' shelves for the perfect moisturizer to combat dehydrated skin. One doesn't exist. Your solution lies elsewhere—in your lifestyle.

Moisture Deprivation

To solve the problem of dehydration, you first need to know what's causing it. Something—perhaps several things—in your environment, health situation, or lifestyle is making your skin dry. Some of the causes listed here are simple to correct, and some take more effort.

- Not enough water intake. You need to drink at least eight glasses, or 64 ounces, of water every day. This is in addition to other beverages you drink during the day, such as tea, coffee, or juice. You may want to eliminate these other beverages entirely, as these beverages can further dehydrate your skin and contribute to other skin conditions, such as acne.

- Forced-air home or office heating and cooling systems. These systems keep the atmosphere dry, which removes moisture from your skin. Use room humidifiers to keep air moist. If you can afford it, install a humidifier on your home furnace. The cost starts at about $350.00 and goes up from there. If you use room humidifiers, make sure you clean them every week so that mold and fungus don't grow in them. Circulating moist mold and fungus in the air can create even more health problems.

◆ Living in a dry climate, such as Colorado, Alaska, Utah, Arizona, and elsewhere. You can't make the air outside more humid, but you can use humidifiers indoors. Fill a pottery crock with water and place several around your house. Refill when the water has evaporated.

◆ Overuse of exfoliants. This dries out skin, making it rough and red. Use your exfoliant less frequently. Use a very light touch with scrub exfoliants, and only use the kind with polyurethane beads or cornmeal.

◆ Overuse of topical prescription medications for skin, such as Retin-A, benzoyl peroxide, or *hydroquinone*. They can make skin dry, red, and inflamed. Cut back on use to every other day or every third day until your skin normalizes and redness is healed.

◆ Using the wrong daily skin care products (cleanser, toner, and moisturizer). First, check to make sure you're using products that harmonize best with your skin type. See Chapters 3 and 4 for specifics. If you feel they're too drying or you experience flaking, check with the sales consultant or skin technician. He or she may ask you to make modifications to your ritual or suggest making product changes. For, example, you may want to switch from a gel to a lotion cleanser.

◆ Using foundation or powder that is too drying for your skin. If your skin feels tight at midday, consider switching your foundation or powder to one with more moisture and less oil-absorption.

> **Clarifying Words**
>
> **Hydroquinone** is a prescription-only topical medication that is used as an antioxidant and skin lightener.

> **Wrinkle Guard**
>
> Fruit juices can be dehydrating to your skin. A small amount of juice, such as half a cup, or 4 ounces, is probably fine. But in larger amounts, you can trigger a rise in blood sugar and a corresponding increase in insulin levels, which creates inflammation. You'll do your skin a favor by eating the fruit rather than drinking fruit juice.

◆ Frequency of chemical peels. Too many salon treatments are simply too much of a good thing. Back off on the frequency. Every six weeks is often enough, and you may want to reduce visits to the salon for peels even further. Talk with your aesthetician to evaluate if your skin dryness is caused by the frequency of peels, your skin care products, or another factor all together.

◆ Medications. Many kinds of medication can cause dehydration. Find ways to get off the medication. If this isn't possible, be sure to take care of the other causes listed here and properly follow all the steps of your daily cleansing routine, and your skin should respond well.

◆ Illness. Even the common cold or flu can dehydrate your skin. If you've been through a more challenging illness, such as cancer, the chemotherapy or radiation treatments can dehydrate your skin. Maintain your daily skin care ritual even when you're under the weather.

◆ Pollution. It seems to be just about everywhere these days and, yes, pollution can dehydrate your skin. To remedy, avoid the other triggers in this list, maintain your daily skin care ritual, and exfoliate regularly.

◆ Airplane travel. The air is considerably drier at 30,000 feet, and airlines do nothing to humidify the air. That's your job. Apply moisturizer before your flight. Transfer some toner that contains a humectant into a spray bottle and spritz your face during the flight. You can also use purified water for your spritz. (Aim carefully. The person next to you may not want an unexpected spritz!) Make sure that your toner contains humectants and doesn't contain any alcohol.

◆ Alcoholic beverages. Alcohol is a *diuretic* and draws fluids from the body, lowering the body's water content. When you're hung over after drinking, it's because your body was dehydrated by alcohol. If you have dehydrated skin, it's best to avoid alcoholic beverages.

> **Wrinkle Guard**
>
> When you're spritzing humectants or water in-flight, be sure that you aren't also sipping on wine or an alcoholic beverage. The end result is that you are still dehydrating your skin, regardless of how much spray you use. Other beverages that could cause dehydration are caffeinated beverages because they have a diuretic effect.

> **Clarifying Words**
>
> A **diuretic** is a food, beverage, herb, or drug that causes the body to increase the output of urine, thus drawing moisture from the cells and leaving the body with a reduced water content.

◆ Smoking. Smoking dries out the body both internally and externally. This affects both smokers and people subjected to second-hand smoke. The only solution is to stop smoking.

◆ Sodas. Both regular and diet sodas contain sodium and are acidic. Drinking these results in dehydrated skin. Avoid sodas and increase your intake of purified water. Carbonated water contains dissolved carbon dioxide, which is highly acidic, so avoid other bubbly drinks as well.

- Not enough sleep. Do whatever it takes to get a good night's sleep. Go to bed earlier to ensure a full night's rest, or take an afternoon nap if you can't get all your sleep in at night.

- Daily intake of starches, white sugar, junk food, french fries, potato chips, and more. Follow the food suggestions in Chapter 21 to avoid the condition of dehydration. In the meantime, banish the junk food from your life.

As you read through this list, it's no wonder that so many people complain about dry skin. Many aspects of our modern lifestyle contribute to this annoying skin condition, and only by changing our regular patterns can we avoid it.

Dehydration Begone

After you have made the lifestyle and environmental changes suggested, it's time to go to work on your skin. Follow these suggestions:

- Correcting dehydrated skin begins with faithfully completing your daily skin care ritual. Be sure to cleanse, tone, and moisturize twice a day—morning and evening.

- Next, exfoliate regularly and gently. You need to remove the buildup of dry skin cells and keratinization from your skin. Use gentle AHAs to dissolve dead skin cell buildup. Improve your skin's NMF—Natural Moisturizing Factor—with lactic acid, urea, squalene, glycerine, or urea treatments.

- For a special skin treatment, apply a hydrating mask that stays moist on the skin. Be sure your mask isn't intended to actually dry while on the skin. Masks are discussed in Chapter 5.

- When outdoors, use moisturizer and sunscreen that prevent skin moisture loss.

- Choose a foundation that seals in moisture, such as one that contains silicone, silica, or glyconucleopeptides.

CAUTION

Wrinkle Guard

One of the most common contributors to dehydrated skin is using a cleanser that's alkaline. This is especially true for some bar soaps for facial cleansing. Other types of skin cleansers can also be alkaline. If you suspect your cleanser is drying out your skin, look for one with a pH of less than 7.

Take essential fatty acids, such as those found in fish oil capsules or flax seed oil, every day. Take about 10 capsules or 2 tablespoons. They will make your skin soft and supple. Eat 5 to 10 servings of vegetables and fruits daily, or at least 2 with each meal.

Skin-spiration

You can purchase Emergen-C at health food stores and at many grocery stores in the health food or supplement aisles.

Keep your electrolytes in balance. Electrolytes help regulate the body's hydration levels. Avoid Gatorade, because it's full of sugars and artificial ingredients. Instead, use Emergen-C packets. Mix one in water when you feel dehydrated.

Salon Hydration

A visit to the skin care salon can prove beneficial to correcting dehydration. Ask for a hydrating facial. You'll get a hydrating mask that contains humectants, vitamins, essential fatty acids, and perhaps collagen. The mask doesn't dry on the face but stays moist and is removed with water.

The skin care technician may use steam to add moisture topically, and then apply a healthy oil on top of a moisturizer.

The process is relaxing, but it's doing more than making you feel good. Your skin could look better immediately. With proper at-home maintenance, your skin can stay moist, plump, and radiant.

The Least You Need to Know

- Dehydrated skin, also known as dry skin, is a temporary skin condition that you can correct.

- Our modern lifestyle and environment can cause dehydrated skin.

- Continue to use your regular daily skin care routine and add some special moisturizing masks and treatments.

- Make lifestyle changes to avoid dehydration in the future.

Chapter 15

Sensitized Skin and Immune System Conditions

In This Chapter

- ◆ Caring for sensitized skin
- ◆ Physical and environmental causes of sensitized skin
- ◆ Treating flare-ups
- ◆ Treating psoriasis, seborrhea, and eczema

Perhaps your skin's been doing great for some time now. It functions well, it's smooth, plump, moist, and radiant. And then something happens to change all that, seemingly overnight. Your skin starts getting sensitive.

It feels inflamed. It burns and stings. It's red and it itches. Your skin has become sensitized. Fortunately, sensitized skin is only a temporary condition and can be remedied.

At times like these, your skin is actually communicating with you. It's asking you to stop irritating it so it can calm down and behave. Your mission is to find the source of the irritation and to make the changes necessary for the irritation to go away. Then, your skin wants some soothing and healing treatments.

Vulnerable to Everything

You may not be able to identify sensitized skin by looking at it. Instead, pay attention to how it reacts. It seems to want something, but you're not sure how to treat it to make it happy and soothed.

When your skin is sensitized, it becomes more vulnerable to stress, the environment, and other day-to-day assaults. Whereas before a light spray of cologne in the morning was innocent enough, when your skin is sensitized, that same cologne could make your skin flake or burn.

Even your daily skin routine can cause inflammation and irritation. When you touch your face, it can hurt. The irritation and inflammation that accompany sensitized skin ages the skin and can create wrinkles, lines, and sagging. What's going on?

Somehow your immune system has been overtaxed and doesn't have the ability to muster up defenses to even the simplest challenges. The first task to solving the condition of sensitized skin is to discover the underlying cause and make necessary corrections.

Think of your immune system has having a limited amount of power. It can use only so much power before it's overloaded and can't perform well. Our immune systems are on the alert to heal us from such health conditions as illness, chronic diseases, colds, flu, and allergies. Other factors that can deplete our immune system's effectiveness are chronic or short-term stress, hyperinsulinism, lack of sleep, and inflammation. In Part 5, you'll learn many lifestyle techniques that help to keep your immune system full of power.

Taxing Your Immune System

In our modern, fast-paced world, our immune systems are constantly struggling to keep us healthy. On a day-to-day basis, we're exposed to more disease-causing bacteria and viruses than ever before in the history of humankind. Heating and air-conditioning systems in the home and office circulate them, as well as other irritants, such as pollen, mildew, and molds. Air pollution harbors the same danger, plus known irritants such as carbon monoxide and auto exhaust fumes.

The immune system protects the body from succumbing to disease, and from developing allergic reactions to all sorts of chemicals, pollutants, and

> **CAUTION**
>
> **Wrinkle Guard**
>
> With sensitized skin, use very gentle exfoliation provided that your skin isn't inflamed. When not inflamed, can use fruit enzymes, rice powder, and oatmeal masks.

fragrances. When the body's immune system is overtaxed, it prioritizes the workload. At these times, the immune system considers it far more important to protect your vital organs and your internal health than to take care of your skin.

Skin-spiration _____

If you have sensitive-type skin, you don't necessarily have sensitized skin. Sensitized skin is a temporary condition that occurs in all skin types. If your genetic skin type is sensitive, your skin is naturally sensitive all of the time. Stay consistent with your daily skin care rituals, keep on using gentle exfoliation, and you can keep your skin healthy and looking great. If your skin seems more sensitive than normal, use the recommendations in this chapter.

This is when you develop sensitized skin. Your skin is a reflection of everything that's going on in your body. Any skin condition is a result of the body's overall well-being. When your skin is sensitized, you need to help out your immune system by lightening its workload. Remove the source of the problem.

Sources of Sensitized Skin

When your skin becomes sensitized, read through the following list to help discover the root cause of your skin condition. While we can't list everything that can create a reaction, as you read through, look for similar stresses and immune system depletion that relate to you and your life. Possible sources of sensitized skin are:

- ◆ Allergic reactions to foods you eat infrequently, such as shellfish, or special treats; they may cause hives. Your body's response to the allergic reaction can deplete the immune system temporarily and thus affect the condition of your skin.

- ◆ Allergic reactions to skin care products or cosmetics. This kind of allergic reaction occurs in less than 10 percent of cases. If you've changed products recently, they may be triggering sensitized skin.

- ◆ Contact with plants or some essential oils. Poison ivy is an example of this kind of sensitization, but you can also have a lower-grade reaction to non-poisonous plants and botanical oils.

CAUTION   Wrinkle Guard _____

Be sure to save and file the product labels from your skin care products and cosmetics. If you have an allergic reaction, you may be able to identify the offending ingredient and avoid it in the future.

◆ New detergent or body soap. If you suspect these, take them back to the store for a refund or else toss them out and buy another brand or another formulation. The allergic reaction can use up some of the power of your immune system and this can affect the condition of your skin. If your immune system is strong, an allergic reaction to a new detergent is unlikely to affect your skin. But this added to other stressors can give you sensitive skin.

◆ Sinusitis. An infection in your sinuses can sap your immune system's defenses.

◆ Asthma. Having asthma indicates an immune system that is already overextended.

◆ Steroids. Prescription medications with steroids block an overactive immune system, but can also stress your body and skin.

◆ Contact with metals, especially nickel. Wearing jewelry made with a nickel alloy can sensitize skin.

◆ Bubble baths, bath salts, and fragrances. These could also promote yeast infections, depending on what skin comes in contact with these products.

◆ Preservatives used in products applied topically and in ingested food products.

◆ Antihistamines and other over-the-counter medications.

◆ The usual suspects—caffeinated beverages, alcoholic beverages, illegal drugs, and smoking.

◆ Sun exposure. Yes, even though this feels great and some people think a tan looks great, sun exposure taxes your immune system. It's trying to prevent those free radicals from harming the body.

> **Wrinkle Guard**
>
> Ted broke out in hives all over his face after eating a Christmas treat. He loved the taste of the candies—dried cherries wrapped in milk chocolate and coated with red coloring. He knew from past experience that he didn't react to chocolate or cherries, so he figured the red-food coloring triggered his hives. Fortunately, it's easy to stay away from red food coloring.

◆ Lack of sleep. Your immune system requires about eight hours of sleep a night to function correctly. You may require less or more, but be sure to get the amount of sleep you need every night.

◆ Hormonal imbalances. These may occur premenstrually or during menopause, or, for men, during middle age. This can sensitize your skin.

◆ Thyroid imbalances. This can sensitize your skin. When the thyroid is either under- or over-producing, the body is out of balance. One side effect is sensitization in general and specifically, of the skin.

◆ Diabetes. This is especially true if you aren't controlling your blood sugar levels with diet and exercise. If needed, use medications. Elevated blood sugar levels cause inflammation. With elevated blood sugar levels, the body's cells aren't getting the glucose they need for health.

◆ Surgery of any kind. Anesthesia, painkillers, and medications need to be detoxified by the liver. This takes priority over detoxing the skin and body from normal daily detoxification. When the body has too many toxins, your skin becomes sensitized. It can take several months for your skin to fully recover from the effects of surgery. This includes cosmetic surgery.

◆ Medications. Any kind of medication, especially prescription medications. These include Retin-A, Accutane, Differin, antibiotics, prednisone, diabetic medications, and blood pressure medications. Medications tax the body's detoxification system, especially the liver. As stated previously, all toxins are processed through the liver. Your liver can become too overburdened to process all toxins efficiently. When the liver gets backed up, toxins can be sent to the skin for excretion. This makes your skin sensitive and perhaps, congested.

◆ Illness. Colds, flu, and more serious diseases can sensitize the skin. So can autoimmune diseases, such as multiple sclerosis, fibromyalgia, arthritis, or cancer.

◆ Chronic stress. Ongoing day-to-day stress with no relief in sight increases cortisol levels, which causes anxiety and depression. It also depresses the immune system, making it more susceptible to disease.

Anything that taxes the immune system or blocks its functioning can give you sensitized skin. As best you can, eliminate the source of the problem. Sometimes you can't, as with elective cosmetic surgery or the use of medications. In those situations, you can take actions to improve your sensitized skin.

CAUTION Wrinkle Guard _____

Jodi loves the islands and spends lots of time in the Caribbean. On each trip, she gets sun poisoning, and has an intense allergic reaction to sand flea bites. She enjoys multiple cocktails every day at a cabana on the beach and spends plenty of time tanning in the sunshine. She returns home a mess. She's fatigued, her skin hurts, sags more, has odd pigmentations, and new wrinkles. The combination of alcoholic beverages and heavy sun exposure taxes her immune system, resulting in the sun poisoning and the allergic reaction to sand fleas. The solution? Avoid the islands, avoid the alcohol, or both. Use heavy-duty sun protection and don't even think about trying to get a suntan.

Treating Sensitized Skin

The commonsense rule of thumb when treating sensitized skin is this: Less is best. When your immune system has too much to deal with, doing less gives both your immune system and your skin an opportunity to rebuild and grow stronger. By doing less, you are cutting back on any activity that can increase your stress load.

Continue your regular daily skin care ritual twice a day. Be extra gentle with exfoliation, as it may be too strong for your skin in its sensitized state.

Use calming and soothing masks, such as an aloe vera, allantion, tea tree oil, or green tea compress. Other soothing ingredients for masks or compresses include licorice and red raspberry.

Take antioxidant supplements, such as alpha lipoic acid and Vitamins C and E. Increase your intake of vegetables and fruits, as they contain healing antioxidants. Take at least 2 tablespoons of essential fatty acids to support the skin and connective tissue. Avoid taking new medications and, where possible, ease off of other medications.

Eat foods that are good *immune system modulators*, such as garlic, seaweed, vegetables, and fruits. Also included are vitamin and trace element supplements.

At the spa, ask your skin care technician for lymph drainage or cold marble stone therapy, as well as treatment with soothing cool mists. More about cold marble stone therapy and lymph drainage are discussed in Chapter 13.

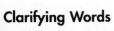

Wrinkle Guard

Be cautious when using new products on sensitized skin. You could get another reaction. Even very soothing products could upset your skin. Go slow, adding only one new product at a time. When in doubt, do a patch test on the inside of your arm to determine if you'll react to the new product.

Clarifying Words

Immune system modulators are foods and supplements that strengthen the immune system. They modulate the immune system so that it's neither overactive, which can lead to autoimmune diseases, nor underactive, which can lead to bacterial and viral infections.

Skin Diseases

Three common skin diseases that require special understanding and treatment are psoriasis, seborrhea, and eczema. In this section, we discuss each one and give you information on how to improve your situation. Be sure to consult with your dermatologist if you suspect you have any of these skin diseases.

Psoriasis

Psoriasis is a chronic and recurring skin disease. It's characterized by a heavy buildup of dead skin cells. What happens is that new skin cells grow so quickly that your skin isn't able to shed the dead cells fast enough to keep up with the growth.

The average healthy skin cell matures in 21 to 28 days. With psoriasis, the skin cells mature in three to six days. The heavy buildup of dead skin cells forms a scaly mass with papules underneath. The skin becomes inflamed and may ooze.

Psoriasis is most common on the elbows, knees, scalp, and chest. It's estimated that over seven million people in the United States have psoriasis. Both men and women get psoriasis and the onset can occur at any age.

Psoriasis is thought to be an immune system disorder in which the immune system becomes overly active. This triggers inflammation, causing the skin cells to grow too quickly.

Many remedies are available for psoriasis. Start with the simpler approaches and move up to the more complex should the simple ones not prove effective. Be sure to consult with your dermatologist before you start any program for psoriasis.

Simple treatments include:

- Natural sunlight. Often clears psoriasis. The ultraviolet protection suppresses the skin's immune response. Get regular daily doses of sunlight, but be sure to use sunscreen to avoid sunburn, which can make the psoriasis worse. For cloudy days, you can purchase skin therapy light boxes that come with special goggles and a timer.

- Coal tar in such forms as shampoos, lotions, and creams. Widely available at drugstores and discount chains. Use caution if you combine coal tar with sunlight. Coal tar can make the skin more vulnerable to sunlight, and therefore, can lead to sunburn or sun damage.

- Anthralin. A topical prescription medication that inhibits cell production, Anthralin can cause irritation on the surrounding skin and stains clothing.

- Topical corticosteroids, or cortisone. These can initially be very effective at reducing skin buildup, inflammation, and itching. Possible side effects include burning, irritation, dryness, acne, and thinning of the skin. Use for a while to get psoriasis under control, but over time, your body develops resistance to these medications and psoriasis can return when you discontinue use.

- Glycolic acid. Excellent at removing dead skin cell buildup. Be sure to use a 1.8 to 3 percent solution with a pH that is no higher than 3.5.

Your dermatologist can advise you on systemic treatments for psoriasis. Most medications are significant drugs that can have serious side effects. Many of the newer treatments include drug therapy with exposure to UVA light. Use these therapies only if other safer methods are ineffective.

For more information on psoriasis and to keep up to date on new treatments, log on to www.psoriasis.org, the website of the National Psoriasis Foundation.

Seborrhea

Seborrhea is a disease of the sebaceous glands. It can be mistaken for acne and blackheads, but the identifying characteristic of seborrhea is increased oil production with scaly, thickened skin. The oil is often thick and sticky. Like acne, seborrhea results in whiteheads, blackheads, and pimples.

Seborrhea occurs on the scalp, sides of nose, eyebrows, behind the ears, and in the middle of the chest. In infants, it's known as "cradle cap." Seborrhea can occur on almost any part of the body or face.

Seborrhea is caused by yeast that's present in the hair follicle. You can control the growth of seborrhea, but it can recur from time to time. Consult a dermatologist if you have more than mild symptoms.

Over-the-counter remedies include dandruff shampoos and ointments that include such ingredients as coal tar, zinc pyrithione, ketaconazole, and selenium sulfide. Sunlight has also been shown to be an effective treatment.

Skin-spiration

You can try home remedy for seborrhea that's often effective. At the health food store, purchase a "greens" powder, such as GreensPlus. The greens powder is a combination of plant foods. Twice a day, mix 1 tablespoon in a glass of water and drink up. You may find that your seborrhea diminishes. Even if it doesn't, the greens drink provides you with plenty of healthful antioxidants, vitamins, and minerals, plus intestinal bacteria support.

You can also ask you dermatologist if an antifungal prescription medications would help control your seborrhea. Prescriptions include topical 1 percent ciclopirozolamine in a cream base, metronidazole, and the oral medication terbinafine.

Eczema

Eczema is also known as atopic dermatitis. Virtually anything can trigger dermatitis. Eczema is a reaction to something you touch or that touches you. As best you can, identify the source of your eczema and eliminate it.

Eczema can appear anywhere on the body. What differentiates eczema from other skin reactions is that it itches and you'll want to scratch. Don't. If you do, you could make the situation worse. Other characteristics of eczema are skin surfaces that are cracked, blistered, crusted, weepy, reddened, patchy, and dry.

The condition is an abnormal response of the body's immune system. Your immune system, in a sense, overreacts to the trigger. Rather than just sending a scout to check out what's going on, your immune system sends in an entire army to annihilate a single and minor offender. The overreaction shows up on your skin as a full-blown and highly uncomfortable rash, irritation, and inflammation.

You must get your immune system back in order to prevent flare-ups in the future. Look to internal solutions first, then move on to topical preparations and, if needed, prescription medications.

Strengthen and boost your immune system with the following foods and supplements:

- Take at least 2 tablespoons of essential fatty acids a day, either in the form of an EFA oil or fish oil capsules. Purchase EFAs at the health food store or at a discount chain. If your eczema is highly troublesome, double the amount to 4 tablespoons. You can't go wrong taking essential fatty acids.

- Take plenty of B vitamins. We recommend liquid B vitamins to assure complete absorption. Liquid B's are absorbed by the mucous membranes of the mouth and aren't digested in the stomach. If you are experiencing lots of stress, your stomach digestion is inefficient. You can use regular B vitamins in capsules or tablets normally, but when your skin is highly stressed, liquid B's are more readily assimilated in the body.

- Often eczema reactions are acidic, so make your body slightly alkaline. Drink a greens drink, such as Greens Plus, twice a day. Just mix the powder in water and drink. It's available at the health food store. Alka Seltzer Gold is great also. It doesn't contain over-the-counter medications, just sodium citrate and potassium citrate. Don't use this everyday, as it isn't nutritive. The greens drink contains valuable antioxidants you need to assist your immune system, but Alka Seltzer Gold is great to keep in your briefcase or handbag for when you really need it.

◆ For supplementation, take a general vitamin and mineral product. You may benefit from taking a trace mineral product which contains approximately 72 trace elements that your body needs in very minute amounts.

◆ Take a dietary supplement that contains special immune system modulators, such as beta glucan, or glyconutrients.

◆ Drink green tea or black tea two to three times a day. The tea contains antioxidants and nerve soothers. The effectiveness of the tea could be the antiallergic properties of tea polyphenols. This suggestion may or may not work for you, but it's worth a try.

Some topical ointments and moisturizers for eczema may offer relief and healing. Use products containing essential fatty acids. Ingredients that have EFAs include triglycerides, linoleic acid, borage oil, primrose oil, fish oil, flaxseed oil, coconut oil, palm oil, and oleic acid.

Use a sun block every time you go outside. Sun blocks contain zinc oxide or titanium dioxide. Avoid chemical sunscreens that contain such ingredients as avobenzone, because they can trigger new flare-ups.

Visit your dermatologist for his or her recommendation for topical ointments or oral medications. Topical corticosteroids—cortisone creams—are most often prescribed. They work great for temporary relief, but they have serious side effects, such as thinning and deterioration of the skin. Cortisone creams can stop being effective after a time, so use them when you need them, but don't use constantly or for long periods of time.

The Least You Need to Know

◆ Sensitized skin is a temporary condition that can be corrected by eliminating the cause of the skin disturbance.

◆ Be very gentle and loving with sensitized skin, continuing your daily ritual and use cooling treatments.

◆ Sensitized skin is an immune system response characterized by inflammation and redness.

◆ Psoriasis, seborrhea, and eczema are relieved through diet and lifestyle changes, plus medical attention.

Chapter 16

Sun-Damaged Skin

In This Chapter

- ◆ Avoiding sun-damaged skin
- ◆ Correcting past sun mistakes
- ◆ Recognizing skin cancer
- ◆ Using self-tanners and bronzers

You've heard it through the grapevine. You've read it in the newspaper. You've seen it on TV, on cable, on the news, and on the Internet. And you're going to hear it again right here. The sun damages your skin. But, more than that, the sun *ruins* your skin.

And yet, despite all the warnings, many people aren't monitoring their sun exposure and certainly aren't using adequate sun protection. Why? Because we get mixed messages all over the place. Swimsuit catalogues don't show sparkling, alabaster-skinned models in skimpy bikinis. Instead, they present models who are heavily tanned blondes and redheads. Blondes and redheads are the people who are at the highest risk for sun damage and skin cancer. But people of all colors and skin tones are susceptible to sun damage and skin cancer.

One of the most predominant cultural images of health is of people who have a highly tanned face and body. They look relaxed, affluent, and popular. The picture doesn't show them 20 or 30 years later with sagging skin, a face full of wrinkles, and multiple scars from sun-cancer procedures and surgeries.

In this chapter, you'll learn how sun exposure can ruin your skin, and how to do the best you can to repair it. You'll learn how to apply sunscreen and how to check for skin cancer. And we hope you learn that natural skin undamaged by the sun's tanning rays can be truly beautiful and healthy looking.

History of Tanning

Sporting a tan wasn't always a sign of living the good life. In fact just the opposite was true in the 1800s when most people were out-of-doors laborers and farmers. Their tans meant that they had lower social and economic status. In those days, the well-to-do and wealthy eschewed time in the sun and preferred the very pale look, indicating they were members of the wealthier class.

In the early 1900s women who lived in the South never went outside without hats and gloves. About that time, more and more people began working inside as the Industrial Revolution gathered steam. The laborers no longer worked outside. They grew pale.

That's when sporting a tan became a status symbol. A tan broadcasted the message that the person had plenty of leisure time to spend outdoors and a higher social status. The prestige of a tan holds true even up to today when we know that tanning can ultimately kill us. Even if a person doesn't get skin cancer, the skin wrinkles and sags prematurely due to sun damage.

Needless to say, skin cancer isn't a status symbol. Neither are wrinkles and sagging. We intellectually know that tanning is a dumb thing to do. But that hasn't changed our preference for a supposedly "healthy" looking tan.

Fortunately, the tide is beginning to shift. Pale skin is "in." Real tans are out. Fake tans are possible. You can choose to be pale one day, and fake-tanned the next—all without damaging your skin and risking skin cancer or worse.

> **Skin-spiration**
>
> To get a sense of the aging effects of sun exposure, look at a part of your body that isn't exposed to the sun, such as your buttocks. Then compare them to the skin on your hands or face. The differences in texture, wrinkles, pigmentation, and elasticity are all due to photo-aging, or sun exposure.

All About Sunshine

The sun greets us when we awaken in the morning and calls us to rest as it sets. The timing of our daily activities, such as waking, sleeping, and eating, are modulated by our circadian rhythms, and those are based on the sun. We need the sun for survival and sustenance.

The sun gives us health bonuses. Sunshine prevents the debilitating disease rickets because it works with the body to produce vitamin D, a necessary vitamin for health. In moderate doses, sunshine can heal immune system skin disorders, such as psoriasis and seborrhea. Your eyes need about 15 to 20 minutes of indirect sunshine a day for your hormones to function properly.

At the same time, the sun can destroy our health. Exposure to the sun causes the formation of free radials on our skin. Free radicals are incomplete molecules that savage the electrons they need from other molecules, thus damaging the other molecules. They damage collagen and elastin, among others. Free radical damage leads to skin damage, aging, wrinkles, and skin cancer.

We need enough sun to be healthy, yet too much sun can make us look old before our time and can even kill us.

The sun radiates three kinds of light:

◆ UVA is the most plentiful type of solar radiation and causes skin damage and skin cancer. UVA can penetrate glass, so you can even get too much sun from sitting in a car or near a sunny window. UVA doesn't feel hot and doesn't burn your skin.

◆ UVB is stronger than UVA and can cause instant skin damage by causing a blistering sunburn.

◆ UVC is filtered out by the earth's ozone layer. However, as the earth's ozone layer continues to be depleted, more UVC radiation reaches the earth. It's also damaging to the skin.

All solar radiation produces free radicals and all solar radiation can give you sunburn, skin damage, and potentially skin cancer.

> **Body of Knowledge**
>
> You've received over 80 percent of the sun's radiation you'll receive in your lifetime by the time you reach your mid-twenties. Yes, sun protection for children is critical. Over 78 percent of all sun exposure is unintentional and comes when driving the car, taking out the garbage, walking the dog, or car-pooling your children.

In addition, all skin types and all skin colors can experience sun damage. So whether your skin is very fair, or very dark, you need sun protection.

Free Radicals

Today we know that virtually all aging is the result of the activity of free radicals. Free radicals occur naturally in the body.

Technically, free radicals are atoms or molecules that are missing one or two of their electrons. In an effort to regain those electrons, they take them from another atom or molecule. When the free radical is successful, it damages its victim by breaking up its chemical bonds. This scavenging of electrons has a snowball effect, leaving chaos and damage in its wake.

Wrinkle Guard

To get a sense of the power of free radicals, cut open an apple and let it sit exposed to the air for 30 minutes. In that time, the apple will turn brown. The browning is caused by oxidation of the exposed surface of the apple. The same type of chemical reaction happens to your skin when exposed to the sun without the benefit of sunscreen.

Most free radicals are derived from oxygen and are known as "reactive oxygen species." Just as we require sun for life, and yet sun can be damaging, so too with oxygen. We need oxygen to breathe and to metabolize food for energy. But oxygen can damage our cells and harm us as well.

Free radicals damage far more than your skin. They're implicated in many health-related issues such as learning disabilities, heart disease, cancer, and Alzheimer's. What neutralizes them are antioxidants. Many cosmeceuticals are antioxidants, and fruits and vegetables contain a wide variety of these powerful nutrients. Keep on eating those vegetables and fruits.

Free Radical Skin Damage

The sun damages our skin by creating a massive amount of free radicals on the surface of the skin. These free radicals damage the molecules of collagen and elastin.

The damaged collagen begins to deteriorate and, in essence, becomes deformed. Healthy collagen is smooth and supple. The more free radical damage you have, the more sagging and wrinkles. The weathered skin you see on people who spend a lifetime in the sun is the result of cross-linked collagen.

Elastin is the protein in your skin that gives it elasticity. Free radicals turn elastin into something resembling a dried-out rubber band. Your skin loses the ability to spring back. The suppleness diminishes and you look aged.

Free radicals also damage melanin production. Melanin is the pigment that gives your skin its color. When melanin production is disrupted, you develop uneven blotches of color in your skin. These blotches can range from simple freckles to big brown blotches. Your pigment production becomes disorderly and unpredictable and eventually your skin will look older.

> **CAUTION**
>
> ## Wrinkle Guard
>
> Some foods and medications can increase the photosensitivity of your skin. Avoid alcoholic beverages, limes, and other citrus drinks on the days you plan to be out in the sun. If you use AHAs, BHAs, or Retin-A, either avoid the sun altogether, or apply a sunscreen with an SPF of 30 over the sunscreen you put on after washing your face in the morning before venturing outside. Wear a hat that protects your face from the sun. Many prescription medications can make your skin more sensitive to the sun, so check the label and read the side effects before venturing outside.

Because of sun exposure and free radicals, your skin cell production actually slows down. In healthy skin, the cells turn over every 21 to 28 days, so there are always plenty of healthy cells to replenish the natural die-off of cells. Sun-damaged skin slows down new cell production. This isn't good. The cells that die off naturally after 21 to 28 days aren't being replaced quickly enough with plump healthy cells. Instead, the skin is filled with dried-up old cells.

The effects of free radicals are shocking. They can make you look way older than your chronological age. And yet we continue to promote the myth that a tan is youthful and healthy.

Massive amounts of free radicals on your skin due to repeated sun exposure cause such a breakdown in normal cell growth and replenishment that this mechanism can go haywire. That's when skin cancer starts. The cells start growing too fast, resulting in skin growths and, ultimately, disease.

> **CAUTION**
>
> ## Wrinkle Guard
>
> If you've ever had even one sunburn in your entire life, you are more susceptible to skin cancer. The cancer shows up on your face many years after the initial sunburn. This is why even children need daily application of sunscreen to protect them from burns today that can turn into skin cancer years from now.

Tanning Booths

Don't even think of going to the tanning booth. They aren't safe. Use of tanning booths is causing an increase in the incidence of skin cancer. No matter what the salesperson tells you, you can get sun damage and skin cancer from the tanning booth. No amount of sunscreen will help.

If you go to the tanning booth in the winter to alleviate the doldrums of lack of sun or to ease the discomfort of SAD—seasonal affective disorder—save your money. Use your saved money to purchase a Light Box. A Light Box is about the size of a laptop computer. It puts out very bright and safe light. By sitting in front of the Light Box for 20 to 30 minutes a day, you can lighten your mood and save yourself from sun damage and the risk of skin cancer. Light Boxes available at www.gaiam.com.

Enter Sunscreens

Daily use of sunscreen protects you from solar radiation. Yes, the sun can still shine on your skin, but the sunscreen blocks the UVA and UVB rays from reaching your skin and creating free radicals.

Sunscreens also prevent your skin from burning and tanning. If you want to have a tan, you still need to apply sunscreen. You can also fake a tan with new self-tanning products and cosmetic bronzers.

Self-tanning products and bronzers usually don't offer sun protection. If they do, you'll find an SPF rating on the container. Don't forget that you need sunscreen when you use bronzers or self tanners.

The *SPF* rating on your sunscreen, moisturizer, and foundation lets you know how long you can stay in the sun without burning. Here's how it works. First of all, you need to know how long you can stay in the sun before your skin gets red. Let's say that's 10 minutes. If you apply a sunscreen with an SPF of 15, you can stay in the sun 10 times 15, or 150 minutes, or two-and-one-half hours before burning. You need to reapply your sunscreen within two-and-one-half hours to have continual sun protection.

If you're not sure how long you can stay in the sun while wearing an SPF of 15, be sure to err on the side of caution. Reapply your sunscreen between every one and a half to two hours.

Clarifying Words

SPF means Sun Protection Factor. All sunscreens are currently labeled with an SPF that lets you know how long you can stay in the sun before burning. Wear a sunscreen with an SPF of 15 or more to get adequate sun protection.

Here's the catch. SPF is only measured for UVB radiation, and not for UVA. You need protection from both. The ingredients that protect you from UVA radiation are avobenzone, titanium dioxide, and zinc oxide. If your sunscreen doesn't contain any of these ingredients, don't bother using it. Toss it out and purchase a product that contains both UVA and UVB protection.

Wrinkle Guard

Both titanium dioxide and zinc oxide sunscreens can be thick and heavy, meaning they create a barrier on the skin. This is good for preventing sun damage, but can be challenging if you have oily or acne-type skins. Be sure to wash your face every evening to remove the sun product. You may need to use exfoliants more frequently if you are reapplying the sun block often throughout the day.

Sunscreens, by definition, use chemicals to prevent sun from harming the skin. Sun blocks contain a physical barrier that keeps the sun's radiation from ever reaching your skin. The two sun blocks that block both UVB and UVA are zinc oxide and titanium dioxide. These two ingredients are less likely to cause allergic reactions than chemical sunscreens. They're found in most foundations and many moisturizers that contain sunscreens.

Applying Sunscreen

You don't want to burn, but you also don't want to tan. Even a light tan is sun damage. You want to stay pale. So make sure you use plenty of sunscreen.

Don't follow the motto of "a little goes a long way." Just the opposite is true: "More is better." Slather it on. Use plenty. In a sense, you can't overdo the application. Rub it in. Reapply every couple of hours, based on the product's SPF and your skin's needs.

Apply to yourself, your spouse, your children, and anyone else who's standing around. Everyone needs sunscreen. Don't be overly confident that you won't burn. The sun isn't forgiving of your errors.

Body of Knowledge

The FDA recommends at least one ounce of sunscreen per application. That means that an 8-ounce bottle will last for eight applications. If you're sharing a bottle, you and your partner each have 4 applications. If you're on the beach all day and you reapply 4 times, you and your partner go through an 8-ounce bottle every day. Also, check the expiration date. If it's out of date, toss it out.

View waterproof and water-resistant sunscreens with some skepticism. Regardless of the SPF rating, most waterproof sunscreens are good for about 80 minutes before they need to be reapplied, and water-resistant sunscreens are good for about 40 minutes. Reapply, reapply, reapply. Nothing ruins a beach or skiing vacation faster than having to deal with deeply sunburned skin. Ouch!

> **CAUTION**
>
> **Wrinkle Guard**
>
> Steven loved to play golf and was completely faithful to careful application of sunscreen on his face, nose, back of neck, and his ears. But he never applied sunscreen to the sides and front of his neck. You guessed it, after years of playing golf, skin cancer appeared on the front side of his neck. The lesson: Splurge on sunscreen and apply to every possible exposed surface.

Be sure to use extra sunscreen and to take along plenty when you plan to be outdoors. Activities such as going to the beach, swimming, hiking, skiing, golfing, tennis, and even gardening require vigilance and reapplication.

Be sure to cover every spot of your face with a sunscreen specially formulated for the face. These sunscreens are usually gentler and more suited to facial wear. Don't forget the back of your neck, the tips of your ears, and your neck. You can reach these areas easily with a spray, stick, or mineral powder sunscreen.

You can use a less expensive sunscreen for the rest of your body. Make sure the SPF is 15 or over. Discard sunscreen if you haven't used the product in six months. Old sunscreen isn't worth using.

Clothing as Sunscreen

Many outdoor clothing retailers sell clothing with SPF ratings. A wide-brimmed sun hat with an SPF of 33 really delivers. No, sunscreen isn't applied to the fabric, but the fabric is very closely woven and actually blocks out the sun's rays.

You can also purchase shorts, slacks, and shirts with SPF. If you are outdoors frequently, this can be a great solution. You won't need to apply sunscreen to areas that are already clothed.

However, if your outdoor wear is made from loosely woven clothing, it may not give you much, if any, sun protection. Our beloved worldwide favorite, blue jeans, offers an SPF of only 8.

So, if you plan to be out in the sun for a significant length of time, apply sunscreen under your clothes.

Also, don't rely on an umbrella to keep off the sun's damaging rays unless the fabric has an SPF. You can get a major burn sitting under an umbrella. Also, if you're sitting on the beach under an umbrella, you can easily burn from the sun's rays reflected off the water and sand.

Reversing Sun Damage

Many of us wish we could turn back the clock and rewrite our younger years. We would have avoided hanging out at the pool or beach. We would have worn sunscreen constantly. We would have pretended that being a pale-skin was hip. Alas, those days are gone and over and we can't undo our misspent sunbathing hours.

However, there are some things you can do to help reverse sun damage.

- Increase the amount of antioxidants in your diet. Eat more fruits and vegetables; add more herbs and spices to your cooking.

- Apply antioxidants directly to your face. Such cosmeceuticals as alpha lipoic acid and DMAE are thought to rebuild collagen and elastin. More research needs to be done to actually prove this, but many people see visible results.

- Stimulate the skin with lymphatic massage or with daily splashing. Use warm water and splash your skin 30 times twice a day before toning. It's thought that the mild stimulation of the water helps the skin heal itself, and it adds moisture.

- Take 2 tablespoons or more of essential fatty acids every day, or take the equivalent in about 10 capsules of fish oil. Yes, you've read this many times by now in this book. Essential fatty acids make a big difference in the quality of your skin.

Skin-spiration

Many of the current crop of glamorous movie stars are staying out of the sun and out of the tanning booth. We applaud their wisdom, and we appreciate their setting a good example for the rest of us. Stars like Nicole Kidman and Rene Zellweger are among the many actresses who seem pleased with their natural skin coloring, while appearing beautiful and radiant.

- Apply a vitamin-based cosmeceutical to your face. It could include vitamins A, C, and E, plus selenium and CoQ-10. You can also find an antioxidant nutritional supplement and take it orally. In this case, what works well on your skin can also work well inside your body.

- Consider microdermabrasion or laser resurfacing that can rebuild collagen and elastin and soothe pigmentation. A face-lift can eliminate sagging.

◆ Retin-A rebuilds collagen and elastin and can reverse sun damage. See your dermatologist if you would like to use this prescription medication.

◆ Some pigmentation can be reversed and will be discussed in Chapter 17.

Keep in mind that while you are attempting to reverse sun damage, you need to be sure to carefully manage your sun exposure wisely. Use protective clothing such as wide-brimmed hats and wear sunscreen daily.

Skin Cancer

Skin cancer is very serious. It can kill you. It is debilitating. And it's preventable. The incidence of skin cancer is growing every year at epidemic levels.

CAUTION

Wrinkle Guard

If you have an unexplained spot, lesion, mole, or discoloration on your skin, go straight to your dermatologist. Don't mess with the spot or pick at it. Have any suspicious spots examined immediately. Early detection is crucial to cure skin cancers.

Over one million new cases of skin cancer are diagnosed in the United States annually. Eighty percent of those will be basal cell carcinoma, 16 percent are squamous cell carcinoma, and 4 percent are melanoma. An estimated 10,250 people will die from skin cancer in the year 2004.

Skin cancer can appear anywhere on the body, but most often in areas that have been exposed to sun radiation. Here's an overview of the three types of skin cancer.

Basal Cell Carcinoma

People who have fair skin, light hair, and blue, green, or gray eyes are at highest risk for basal cell carcinoma. But dark-skinned people are also at risk. This type of skin cancer grows slowly, seldom spreads, and is easily detected. Standard treatments cut off or burn off the carcinoma. A person has a better than 95 percent cure rate if detected and treated early.

The five warning signs of basal cell carcinoma:

◆ An open sore that bleeds, oozes, or crusts and remains open for more than three weeks.

◆ A reddish patch on chest, arms, shoulders, or legs. May itch or hurt, or may not.

◆ A shiny bump or nodule that's translucent. Can be any color, from white, pink, or red to tan, black, or brown. May be confused with a mole.

- A pink growth with a slightly elevated rolled border. Has a crusty center indentation. Tiny blood vessels may develop on the surface.

- A scarlike area with poorly defined borders. Color is white, yellow, or waxy.

If you suspect you have any of these, go to the dermatologist and have it checked out.

Squamous Cell Carcinoma

Squamous cell carcinomas usually appear on sun-exposed areas of the body, but can be found on any area of the body, including mucous membranes. They usually remain localized on the skin, but in a small number of cases, the spread to distant tissue and organs. When this happens, it can be fatal.

Squamous cell carcinomas often occur where skin has been injured, on areas such as burns, scars, and long-term sores, or areas exposed to x-rays or chemicals like arsenic or petroleum by-products. Sometimes the carcinomas appear for no apparent reason and may be genetically inherited.

Fair-skinned individuals are more likely to develop this squamous cell carcinoma. Two-thirds of the skin cancers that dark-skinned individuals of African descent develop are squamous cell carcinomas.

The warning signs of squamous cell carcinomas are

- A wartlike growth that crusts and may bleed.

- A red, scaly patch with irregular borders that bleeds or crusts.

- An open sore that bleeds and crusts for weeks and doesn't heal.

- An elevated growth with a central depression that may bleed and could grow rapidly.

Squamous cell carcinoma has a better than 95 percent cure rate if detected and treated early.

Melanoma

Melanoma is the most serious form of skin cancer. If detected in its early stages, it's usually curable. If the cancer advances and spreads, it's difficult to treat and can be fatal.

In 2004, one person in the United States will die every hour of melanoma, with older Caucasian males suffering the highest mortality rates. The incidence of melanoma among Caucasians has more than tripled between 1980 and 2003. For women between the ages of 25 and 29, melanoma is more common than any other type of cancer. Melanoma accounts for more than 77 percent of skin cancer deaths.

Melanoma originates in the *melanocytes*, where the body's pigmentation is produced. Most melanomas are dark in color, either black or brown, but they can also be devoid of pigmentation, and become skin-colored, pink, red, or purple.

In situ melanoma means that it is localized and hasn't invaded surrounding tissue or other areas of the body. *Invasive* melanomas are those that have spread into the skin tissue and even into other areas of the body. Invasive melanoma is more serious.

Clarifying Words

Melanocytes are the cells that produce the pigment melanin. This pigment colors our skin, hair, and eyes. Melanin is heavily concentrated in skin moles.

Melanomas are usually brown, black, or multicolored patches, or nodules with an irregular outline. They may crust or bleed and often form on top of existing moles.

If a mole changes or you have any odd growths on your body, go immediately to the dermatologist or family doctor. Don't hesitate and don't delay. Skin cancer is serious.

Self-Tanners and Bronzers

Now that you're not going to be sitting in the sun, under a sun lamp, or on the tanning booth table, maybe you're unhappy with how pale you're going to be. Don't fret. You can still look tan. You can fake it with self-tanning lotions and cosmetic bronzers.

The secret to using a self-tanner is in the application. Use a face formulation to tan your face, and a body self-tanner for the rest of your body.

First, exfoliate, wash, and then dry the area to be tanned. Apply in a single thin layer; being careful not to overlap application or you could end up with streaks. Apply when naked. Don't rub up against anything or touch any part of your body while the tanner is working. This means you can't sit down or get dressed until the product is done working—about 15 minutes. Don't exercise, bathe, or swim for at least three hours.

Wash your hands immediately after application. Use a nailbrush to make sure you don't have tanner under your nails. You may need to scrub off your palms with an exfoliant scrub; otherwise you could end up with orange palms.

Reapply every day until you achieve the depth of color you desire. Always apply sunscreen daily. The self-tanners don't offer sun protection.

Your tan will slough off as the skin cells naturally die off and exfoliate. That's OK. To reapply, use the same procedure as before. Just exfoliate, wash, and dry your skin, then reapply. To maintain a self-tan, you may need to reapply every five to seven days.

You can also achieve a tan by going to a self-tanning studio where you pay to be sprayed all over with the tanner. You stand naked or nearly so in a small chamber, use a shower cap, close your eyes, and automatic sprayers—sort of like a car wash—distribute an even amount of tanner all over your body. Wait a couple of minutes, walk out, and dress. Voilà, you are tanned from head to toe.

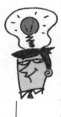

Skin-spiration

Be sure to read the directions for self-tanners very carefully and follow directions. Expect some initial trial and error until you master the application.

Drawbacks include one serious safety and health concern. No one knows how safe it is for you to inhale the spray. You'll hear more about this as research is completed, so stay tuned for news in the future.

Bronzers give you immediate color for both your face and body. They're great if you want to fake a tan on your face and yet be able to wash it off come evening. However, just like mascara and foundation, the bronzer can streak with tears or sweat, and it can rub off on clothing.

Avoid bronzers at the beach or pool—you'll be streaked within hours. But a bronzer can be a nice way to dress up in the summer and go barelegged. The mineral powder bronzers contain an SPF of 15 to 20, depending on the brand. If you use other bronzers, you need to apply sunscreen under your bronzer so you are protected.

The Least You Need to Know

- Any amount of sun exposure can cause skin damage and lead to skin cancer.
- Apply sunscreen every day and keep reapplying as needed.
- Recognize the first signs of possible skin cancer and visit your dermatologist or family doctor immediately.
- Use self-tanners or bronzers if you prefer to look tanned.

17

Pigmentation or Skin Discoloration

In This Chapter

- ◆ Understanding pigmentation problems
- ◆ Getting to the root of the condition
- ◆ Solutions for skin discoloration

The ideal look for healthy skin is even pigmentation. No matter what your skin color, whether dark, light, or somewhere in between, you want a uniformly radiant and luminescent skin color.

Skin pigmentation problems are becoming more and more common. These conditions of uneven color, dark blotches (called hyperpigmentation) or light areas (called hypopigmentation) are distressing. Some conditions that result from hormonal changes or aging can be corrected through topical treatments and making lifestyle changes. Other techniques are available for more stubborn pigmentation problems.

Fortunately, most skin pigmentation disorders don't affect your health, but all such disorders affect the way you look. In this chapter, you'll learn about hyper- and hypopigmentation, their causes, and how to correct the situation.

Spot-Free

The natural pigment in your skin is called melanin and melanin-forming cells are called melanocytes. All skin colors have the same number of melanocytes. The amount of activated melanocytes in your skin determines your basic skin color. Fair-skinned people have fewer activated melanocytes than dark-skinned people. When melanin is deposited in the skin unevenly, with brown, tan, or ash-colored areas, the skin condition of pigmentation occurs.

The skin condition of pigmentation occurs in either light or dark patches on the face and other areas of your body. The condition isn't usually a medical problem, but mostly cosmetic. This means that the condition is harmless, but it doesn't look attractive and can detract from your appearance. A pigmentation condition comes in two colors: red and brown, but the variations can range from tan to very dark brown and pink to dark maroon. The brown comes from melanocytes and the red from blood vessels.

The causes of pigmentation come from both outside the body and from within.

> **CAUTION**
>
> **Wrinkle Guard**
>
> Some changes in skin pigmentation could be an early warning sign of skin cancer. If the skin coloration change seems unusual in any way, visit your dermatologist immediately. For more information on skin cancer, refer to Chapter 16.

Outside Sources of Pigmentation

You can develop pigmentation from the following external situations.

- Freckles and sunburn caused by sun exposure.

- Phototoxic reactions caused by sun exposure after the use of deodorant soaps, scented toiletries, and various cosmetics. These products make the skin more susceptible to the sun's rays and your skin can burn more readily.

- Solar lentigenes, commonly known as age spots or liver spots, usually appear on older skins and result from unprotected sun exposure. They are the result of sun damage and not liver malfunction. On lighter skin, they appear as brown freckles that grow over time. On darker skin tones, solar lentigenes are ashen gray.

- Laser hair removal can leave spots if the laser accidentally burns the skin. This occurs more frequently with darker-skinned people than fair-skinned people, but it can occur in with any skin color.

◆ Scars from wounds, scrapes, stitches, and surgeries. Discolored scars can also result from picking at blemishes.

The pigmentation condition from these external sources can be either *hyperpigmentation*, which is darker than your skin tone, or *hypopigmentation*, which is lighter than your skin tone.

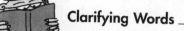

Clarifying Words

Hyperpigmentation is the overproduction of melanin from the melanocytes. **Hypopigmentation** is the failure of melanocytes to produce melanin.

Inside Sources of Pigmentation

Skin discoloration can also be caused by sources within your body or by something you ingested. Here are some sources of pigmentation with suggestions for corrections. They range from mild to serious.

◆ Birth control pills. To correct, talk with your doctor to switch to another product or formulation.

◆ Injected contraceptive preparations. Switch back to birth control pills or use other forms of contraception.

◆ Birth control patch. Switch back to birth control pills or use other forms of contraception.

◆ Pregnancy and nursing. Sometimes called a pregnancy mask, this discoloration fades after nursing and your hormone system returns to normal.

◆ Lupus, an autoimmune disorder. See your doctor for safe suggestions to lighten your skin.

◆ Illnesses and medications. Steroids can cause skin discolorations, as can some other medications. If you suspect your medication, check with your pharmacist or go online to research drug side effects. Ask you doctor to suggest safe ways to lighten skin. Don't discontinue your medication until you have a satisfactory and healthy alternative that's approved by your doctor.

◆ Age. Improve your lifestyle factors per the suggestions in Part 5 of this book. Pay close attention to your diet, sleep habits, and get plenty of exercise.

◆ Birthmarks. Colors range from dark red to brown. Birthmarks can sometimes be removed with laser treatments, and many fade over time. If a birthmark starts to grow and spread, contact your dermatologist immediately.

- Leucoderma, also known as vitiligo, affects 1 to 2 percent of the population and is characterized by depigmented areas. Associated with Addison's disease, diabetes mellitus, pernicious anemia, and thyroid dysfunction, this condition may be a disorder of the immune system. Some patients have antibodies to melanin. If you have leucoderma, avoid sun exposure and wear sunscreen constantly. Topical corticosteroids, such as cortisone cream, may help. Consult your dermatologist for treatment recommendations.

- Albinism is a rare, inherited disorder in which the skin doesn't contain melanin. Avoid all sunlight. Use sunscreen constantly. Wear protective clothing. Don't expose the skin to sun radiation. Because your melanocytes don't produce melanin, you can't tan. You are highly susceptible to skin cancer.

By understanding the cause of skin discoloration, you can find ways to prevent skin discoloration and ways to correct most situations.

Growths That Discolor Skin

Moles, skin tags, and warts are skin growths that also discolor skin. We've included them here and give you guidance for caring for them.

- Moles. These can be light or dark in color. Moles may appear with age, and might be raised or flush with the surface of the skin. Moles must be removed surgically. Never mess with a mole: Don't wax over it and don't pull hair out of a mole. Instead, clip the hair close to the surface of skin. If a mole changes or grows, contact your dermatologist immediately. Your dermatologist can remove warts.

- Skin tags. These often grow on the neck, shoulders, and chest. They can be surgically removed, or you can try dabbing a small amount of salicylic acid at the base of the tag daily until it drops off. They are harmless.

- Warts. Warts are a skin growth with either light or dark pigment. They can be removed surgically, or salicylic acid will kill warts if applied once or twice a day over a longer period of time. Dr. Scholl's Wart Remover works well.

If any of these skin growths change size or color, be sure to check with your dermatologist. They may need to be removed.

Solutions to Skin Discoloration

Virtually all skin hyperpigmentation can be corrected. Some of the solutions take time (as in months), some require a doctor's prescription, and others can be pricey. The following are ways to correct many skin discolorations. If you are currently working with a physician, be sure to ask for advice before making changes. The solutions on the first half of the list are widely available without a prescription.

◆ Stopping birth control pills will reverse skin discoloration, but it may take months for significant improvement. Use camouflage concealer until the skin clears up on its own. Also, be sure you have an alternate and safe birth control method before going off the "pill."

◆ Always use sunscreen to prevent or reduce discoloration.

◆ Avoid skin care products that make your skin photosensitive to the sun. If you suspect a certain product is the source of your problem, stop using it and see if your skin discoloration fades with time.

> **Skin-spiration**
>
> New skin lightening and brightening products regularly become available. Check with your skin care technician or dermatologist to learn about the newest treatments.

◆ AHAs in exfoliants or moisturizers can't lighten skin by themselves. But when used with lightening treatments, such as hydroquinone, kojic acid, or other topical lightening products, they help improve skin's appearance and may help the other treatments better penetrate the skin.

◆ Vitamin C skin serums lighten skin and are highly effective when used with AHAs.

◆ Herbal skin lighteners include licorice, raspberry, bearberry, rice, kiwi, mulberry, grape seed extract, and echinacea. You can find these ingredients on the labels of drugstore and department store skin care products formulated to lighten skin.

◆ Camouflage concealer gives you immediate cosmetic results. Dermablend, which is widely available, is an excellent camouflage concealer. Ask the sales consultant to show you how to apply.

> **Body of Knowledge**
>
> Dark circles under your eyes aren't considered a pigmentation problem. They're caused by lack of sleep, a buildup of toxins within the body, and can be genetic. You can learn how to lighten under-eye circles in Part 5.

◆ Light-diffusing foundation can work miracles to distract the eye from seeing skin discolorations. The foundation doesn't hide or cover up the discoloration, but it makes it much less noticeable.

Consult with your dermatologist about the following solutions:

◆ Bleaching creams such as hydroquinone inhibit formation of new pigment. It takes about 24 days to see a change. Any sun exposure can darken bleached skin, so you need to consistently wear protective sunscreen. If the cream is irritating your skin, cut back the frequency of use.

◆ Laser resurfacing treatments can reduce dark pigmentation, but we don't recommend it. Laser resurfacing is a very serious procedure done only in a doctor's office. Its primary purpose is to correct scarring and wrinkling. One side effect can be hypo- or hyperpigmentation, which is exactly what you're trying to get rid of.

◆ Azelaic acid inhibits melanin production and is effective against acne. It takes several months to see results.

◆ Retin-A and other topical retinoic acids are not effective against discoloration on their own, but they are helpful in combination with hydroquinone or azelaic acid.

Using any of these techniques requires patience and perseverance. But you can achieve a more evenly toned skin. Give yourself and your skin time, love, and the gift of patience.

The Least You Need to Know

◆ Skin discoloration, or pigmentation, is usually a temporary condition if treated.

◆ You can improve the appearance of your skin by first understanding the cause of the condition.

◆ Correcting skin discoloration takes time and patience.

◆ If a skin discoloration appears suddenly or grows, see a dermatologist immediately.

Chapter 18

Premature Aging

In This Chapter

- ◆ How the skin ages
- ◆ Understanding prematurely aged skin
- ◆ Making lifestyle changes
- ◆ Rejuvenating your skin

All skin ages. As we get older, all aspects of our bodies show the effects of age. That's natural. Sure, at times we all wish we could turn back the clock and have youthful-looking skin, but wishes won't make anyone any younger. However, while most of us will long for younger-looking skin as we get older, some of us are wishing for it when we're actually still young.

That's because some people have facial skin that ages prematurely. Even at the age of 25 or 30, their face has way too many "age-inappropriate" wrinkles, and the skin sags and has a dull, coarse, or leathery appearance. Thankfully, premature aging is a skin condition and it can be remedied, making the skin look better with fewer visible signs of aging.

Genetics definitely plays a role in premature aging, but how you live on a day-to-day basis and improper skin care can also bring on early aging. With the new skin-treatment technologies available today, combined with new research information about the causes of aging and how to reverse it, you can actively make a difference in your skin. It can look better and look younger.

In this chapter, you'll learn how to correct the temporary condition of premature aging and what kinds of results you can expect.

How Skin Ages

Skin ages in a multitude of highly complex ways. There are many causes. No one single factor is the main culprit. This is unfortunate, because it would be easier to reverse the effects of aging if you could pinpoint one villain, such as the sun or hormones. Then, you would only need to correct one thing.

Instead, because skin ages synergistically—meaning many factors create a virtual conspiracy to make a person look older—the only effective offense is a good defense. There are two types of aging: intrinsic and extrinsic. Intrinsic aging is genetic—your genes can predict which types of wrinkles you'll have as well as whether your skin will sag a little or a lot. Not much can be done to prevent intrinsic aging. But cosmetic surgery can help.

Extrinsic aging comes from lifestyle factors. These include sun exposure, regular daily skin care, facial expressions, stress levels, eating well or poorly, exercise and more. Fortunately, you can manage your lifestyle to prevent premature again.

But before we get to a good defense, let's discuss the factors that mutually share the responsibility for aging skin.

- Sun damage is an extrinsic aging factor. Sun exposure creates a massive attack of free radicals that cause wrinkling, sagging, and damage to collagen and elastin.

- Pollution is an extrinsic aging factor. The same free radical bombardment is triggered by air pollution on the surface of the skin, and by inhaling the air, drinking the water, etc. Such normal activities of daily life promote free radical damage both internally and to your skin.

- Smoking. Also extrinsic. Smoking is an absolutely terrible way to treat your skin. A trained skin care technician can tell just by looking if you are a smoker or not—your skin tells all. Smoking causes free radical damage which depletes collagen and elastin.

- Genetics is an intrinsic aging factor. Your skin cells may be genetically programmed to slow down replenishment at a younger age than other people.

- Chronological aging. Every year, your skin produces less sebum and has fewer fat cells to keep it plump. Skin is thinner and looks more transparent as we age.

◆ Inflammation. This is caused by many different factors, such as the sun, illness, and pollution. Eating foods high in sugars and refined flours also causes inflammation. Inflammation is also caused by stress and overtaxing the immune system. When a person can eliminate or reduce inflammation, some signs of aging can be reduced.

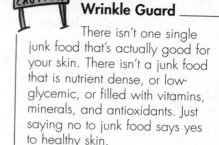

Wrinkle Guard

There isn't one single junk food that's actually good for your skin. There isn't a junk food that is nutrient dense, or low-glycemic, or filled with vitamins, minerals, and antioxidants. Just saying no to junk food says yes to healthy skin.

◆ Hormone imbalances. These include thyroid, pituitary, and adrenal fatigue.

◆ Hormonal depletion. This comes naturally with age, but check out the Fountain of Youth exercises in Chapter 24 to learn how to keep your hormones functioning well as you get older.

◆ Immune system suppression. This is a side effect of some prescription medications, such as steroids and cortisone, and is also caused by ongoing, long-term stress.

◆ Immune system imbalances. Autoimmune diseases, long-term stress, the natural aging process, and an unhealthy lifestyle cause these.

◆ Poor nutrition. A diet heavy on junk food, sugar, starches, and sodas is unhealthy for your whole body, including your skin. Instead, eat vegetables, fruits, meats, and good fats.

◆ Unhealthy lifestyle. Sleep deprivation, too much ongoing stress, and inadequate amounts of relaxation will show up in your skin.

Although you can't do anything about genetics or chronological aging, there's plenty you can do to remedy or reverse most of these aging factors.

Skin-spiration

If you have an autoimmune disease or other chronic conditions, such as diabetes, you can reduce premature aging by following a food plan that eliminates junk foods and refined starches, and instead focuses on eating animal protein with vegetables and fruits. Take Essential Fatty Acids daily. Ask your doctor or health practitioner for more ways to manage and improve your health situation.

Premature Aging

Virtually all premature aging is preventable. The only exception is the genetic component. If you were born with skin predisposed to age early, it will. If you suspect this to be your situation, check with your siblings, mother, father, aunts, and uncles—your whole family. If the family consensus is that they age early, you will, too. But that doesn't mean you can't improve the situation. With regular exfoliation and good daily care, you can make the most of the skin you were born with.

You have the skin condition of premature aging if you feel that your skin looks older than it should. Up until the age of 45 or so, skin is usually supple with a couple of wrinkles and minimal sagging.

Premature aging shows up as wrinkles with tiny fine lines going in all directions, and not just a few lines around the eyes. Some identifying characteristics are skin that's coarse, dull, or leathery. The skin is loose, has deeply colored discoloration or pigmentation, and poor circulation. Poor circulation means that fewer nutrients are getting to the skin for nourishment.

Genetic skin types that are more prone to premature aging are oil-dry skin, which naturally produces less sebum, and sensitive skin, which can either be overly dry or overly oily. While having oily-type skin seems undesirable when a person is young, oily skin becomes a blessing as we age, as oily-type skin ages more slowly than the other skin types.

Although genetics definitely contributes to premature aging of the skin, it isn't the most significant factor. The primary cause of the aging is the activity, food, or lifestyle item you don't want to give up. Whatever bad habit you are desperately hanging on to and refuse to give up is the culprit. You already know what it is. Perhaps it's your sweet tooth, cigarettes, sunbathing, or being a couch potato. Your skin will improve within weeks of giving up your vice. Not giving up these bad habits ensures that your skin will continue to look old before its time. Even if you take drastic actions, such as laser resurfacing, and you don't stop the bad habit, your skin will eventually resort to its former condition.

Amazing Skin

Your skin wants to rejuvenate itself at any age and in any condition. It's one of the truly amazing qualities of skin. No matter how poorly you have treated it, your skin wants to be healthy. Fortunately, there's plenty you can do assist its recovery:

◆ Continue your basic skin care ritual for your skin type with daily cleansing, toning, and moisturizing. Details on the best routine for your skin type are found in Chapter 4.

◆ Exfoliate normally, per your skin type. It's okay to be a bit more aggressive by increasing the number of exfoliations per week by one, or by adding an enzyme peel along with chemical or scrubs, but remember to be gentle with your skin.

◆ Make the lifestyle changes recommended in Part 5. These include generous use of sunscreen and avoiding unprotected sun exposure. Eat low-glycemic foods. Avoid junk food. Avoid starches and sugars. Stay away from all types of sodas. Stay hydrated by drinking plenty of water. Do stress-soothers daily. Use anti-anxiety techniques.

◆ Take nutritional supplements including vitamins, minerals, trace elements, extra B vitamins, and antioxidants. See Part 5 for specific recommendations.

◆ Exercise, lifestyle changes, and hormone therapy can assist with hormonal imbalances. For hormone therapy, you can use progesterone creams and increase the amount of phytoestrogens in your daily diet.

◆ Immune system function can often be improved with diet, relaxation, and other lifestyle changes, such as exercise.

◆ Reduce your stress load. Learn how in Chapter 22.

◆ Detoxify your body. Use the information in Chapter 23.

◆ Reduce inflammation through improving diet, increasing antioxidants, and reducing stress.

◆ Microdermabrasion or laser resurfacing can help clear up some signs of aging and make your skin look refreshed and relaxed.

◆ Plastic surgery can lift sagging skin and smooth wrinkles.

Give your skin time to rejuvenate. In doing so, you'll be doing a favor for your entire body and your overall health. Whenever you make positive changes for your skin, it will positively affect your entire being.

Salon Rejuvenation

A visit with a skin care specialist can get you on the right track to repairing prematurely aged skin. Ask for advice on nutritional supplements that contain antioxidants and revitalizing vitamins and minerals.

The goal of your skin treatment will be to increase cell turnover and make its rate more consistent with that of healthy skin. The rate of healthy skin cell turnover is every 21 to 28 days. Here are some suggestions:

- Rejuvenating facial combines deep cleansing with application of antioxidants and serums designed to reduce the visible signs of aging.

- A glycolic acid peel with vitamin C removes dead skin cells, thoroughly exfoliates the skin, and stimulates new collagen production. New collagen production makes your skin not only appear younger, but also makes it behave as younger skin. Your skin will look more radiant, more vibrant, plump, and smooth.

- Microdermabrasion is also good for thoroughly exfoliating dead skin cells and increasing cell turnover.

These skin treatments need to be repeated every four to six weeks, about as often as skin cells turn over. Your skin won't benefit with only one treatment, so schedule regular professional treatments, or learn how to continue skin treatments at home, per your skin care technician's advice. Otherwise, your results won't last.

The Least You Need to Know

- Premature skin aging may be prompted by genetics, but is most likely exaggerated by bad lifestyle habits.

- You can correct prematurely aged skin by making lifestyle changes and performing regular daily skin care maintenance.

- With some exceptions, the skin condition of prematurely aged skin can be improved and corrected.

- Use laser resurfacing and plastic surgery when other techniques and changes haven't given you desired results.

Part 5

Creating Healthy Skin Through a Healthy Lifestyle

Your skin reflects exactly what's going on inside your body. And there's nothing you can do about it, except to make sure that what's going on inside your body is healthy and noninflammatory. In this part, you'll learn step by step what lifestyle changes to make. First, you'll learn how to manage your sun exposure. Then you'll find out which foods cause inflammation and which ones give your skin a soft and radiant glow. We discuss how to custom-tailor your physical and emotional environment to keep your skin healthy.

We'll tell you how to do simple daily detoxification activities to reduce your body's burden of the toxins that can cloud your skin. We'll also help you develop a routine of physical exercise including aerobics, strength training, and stretching that you do at least three times a week. Your skin will thank you, as will every cell in your body.

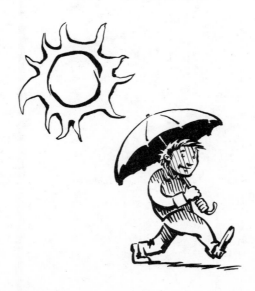

Chapter 19

Menopause

In This Chapter

- Understanding how menopause affects your skin
- Remedying menopause symptoms through lifestyle
- Caring for menopausal skin
- Skin care for aging men

Every woman will go through menopause at some point in her adult life. Many things in her body will change, including her skin. During menopause, the skin becomes drier, it will tend to sag more, and it will either lose or gain pigmentation.

Menopause, including the period leading up to actual menopause, known as perimenopause, can be a challenging time for you and your skin. You'll want to change several aspects of your regular skin care routine. You could need to change skin care products, and start using products that provide more moisture. You'll need stronger or more frequent exfoliation treatments to increase the cell turnover rate.

In this chapter, you'll learn how to care for your skin as it approaches menopause, during menopause, and in the years that will follow. Take heart. Passing through menopause doesn't mean you can't still have radiant and lovely skin.

Hormonal Skin Changes

Menopause is a significant fact of life for every woman. Eventually, all women stop having menstrual cycles and are no longer able to become pregnant. This happens when a woman's hormone production decreases and her body no longer produces adequate amounts of estrogen, a hormone essential for reproduction.

During the three to seven years leading up to menopause, called *perimenopause*, a woman's hormone production is gradually slowing down. With decreased hormone production, the body changes and so does the skin. Like puberty, menopause is a long-term event. It takes time for a woman's menstrual periods to cease and the body to fully change.

Clarifying Words

Menopause is the cessation of menstruation, occurring around the age of 50. A woman is considered to be through menopause when she hasn't had any menstrual cycles for over 12 consecutive months. The age for menopause varies, and generally ranges from about 43 through 59. **Perimenopause** is the three-to seven-year period prior to menopause during which estrogen levels begin to drop.

Skin-spiration

There is no cure for menopause, because it's not a disease. It's a natural fact of life. But there are many ways to stay healthy and vibrant during and after this phase of life, and nothing about menopause means you can't have good-looking skin.

The information in this chapter shows you how to care for your skin through perimenopause, menopause, and beyond. For most women, the change is gradual, allowing you time to adjust your skin care routines as your skin changes. But if a woman has a full hysterectomy in which the ovaries have been removed, she can go through menopause within weeks or days. Also, women who are using the medication tamoxifen as part of breast cancer treatment may experience menopause early and rather suddenly.

Some women breeze through perimenopause and menopause without any symptoms. If this is you, consider yourself lucky. Other women may experience the following symptoms in the years of perimenopause leading up to menopause: hot flashes, irritability, anxiety, depression, irregular menstrual cycles, weight gain around waist, vaginal dryness, night sweats, joint aches and pains, loss of muscle tone and bone mass, lack of coordination, and vertigo.

Here's how your skin changes throughout perimenopause and at menopause:

◆ Loss of muscle mass and muscle tone causes facial skin to sag.

◆ Facial skin gets thinner and seems more translucent.

◆ Skin excretes less oil, becoming drier.

- Skin cells become more compacted—they aren't as plump.

- Skin cell turnover slows, giving skin a dull and tired look.

- With a lower level of oil production, moisture is lost via evaporation from the surface of the skin.

- Collagen production decreases and collagen fibers collapse, making the entire structure of the skin start to sag and loosen.

- The amount of elastin in the skin decreases and stops being well connected within itself, making the skin less elastic.

- Melanin production slows, so a woman's skin tone fades. Some women have increased skin discoloration. A decline in melanin makes a woman more prone to faded spots.

- Glandular activity slows down, meaning that you don't sweat as much. Because you sweat less, your skin doesn't eliminate toxins as readily.

- Your skin is more susceptible to developing skin disorders such as seborrhea, eczema, psoriasis, and rosacea.

What all these changes mean is that your skin becomes drier, more wrinkled, and has less elasticity. Your skin sags more and seems looser. The skin loses thickness and small spider veins that were once virtually invisible become noticeable.

As far as we know, you can't change the fact of menopause or change the timing to later in life. Menopause happens. It's a part of the natural cycle of a woman's life. What you can do is care for your body well during the menopausal years. But don't despair, you are still in charge of how good your skin looks. It doesn't necessarily take more work, but a different focus and modified skin care rituals.

Skin-spiration

Skin care lines now offer products specifically designed for menopausal and post-menopausal women. You'll find ingredients, including cosmeceuticals that promote faster cell turnover and that reduce the appearance of spider veins while helping to increase elasticity and collagen.

Making the Most of Menopause

Taking care of your skin is way more than skin deep. By keeping your entire body vibrant and healthy, you'll be doing the best things possible for your face. What you do for your overall wellness is far more important than what specifically you put on your skin. Of course, what you put on your skin counts, too.

First, let's discuss ways to keep your body vibrant and healthy, as well as ways to keep your hormones functioning properly. Your body excretes more than 57 different hormones. These hormones regulate many bodily functions, such as your digestion, stress reactions, weight gain or loss, and even your sleep.

Reproductive hormones—the ones whose production wanes through menopause, namely estrogen, testosterone, and progesterone—are just a few of your body's hormones. Your other hormones can stay at optimal production throughout your lifetime even if your body has decreased its production of your reproductive hormones. Keep your hormones at optimal levels through exercise and good nutrition. Check out the Fountain of Youth exercises in Chapter 24 that help with hormone balancing.

> **CAUTION**
> **Wrinkle Guard** _____
>
> HRT, or hormone replacement therapy for reducing the effects of menopause, is controversial at this time. Medical research studies have been halted due to an increase in the rate of strokes, breast cancer, and heart disease for women who use HRT. Therefore, we won't discuss the use of HRT in this book. Some doctors believe it's valuable to reduce severe menopausal symptoms. Others recommend it for short-term use. Ask your doctor for his or her recommendations.

The following tips can help ease and reduce negative effects of menopause on your skin and the rest of your body. The more you can keep all of your hormones functioning optimally, the more benefits you'll notice in the condition of your skin. It will be more radiant, plump, and dewy. See Part 5 for more specifics.

- Stay at a healthy weight. Don't get too thin and don't become overweight. It's healthiest to maintain a constant weight over a long period of time and not to have your weight fluctuate frequently.

- Do strength training to maintain muscle mass and tone and to keep body fat levels in the safe range. For women over the age of 50, body fat needs to stay between 20 to 30 percent for optimal health and higher metabolism. Strength training includes using free weights, working out with health club weight machines, or doing Pilates-type exercises. Do one-hour sessions two times a week. Stay strong. Strength training also helps keep your bones dense and healthy.

- Do aerobic exercises at least three times a week for 20 minutes or more. Get your heart rate up. Sweat. Keep your joints agile and functioning properly. This helps avoid osteoporosis.

♦ Take essential fatty acids daily, preferably about 2 tablespoons a day, to help protect against cancer, menopause symptoms, high cholesterol, and bone loss. Essential fatty acids are great for the health of joints, skin, hair, and moods.

♦ Eat 5 to 10 servings of vegetables and fruits daily. Eat for enjoyment, of course, but also for antioxidants, bioflavinoids, vitamins, minerals, and fiber.

♦ Do activities that create inner and outer balance, such as yoga and/or meditation.

♦ Do the Fountain of Youth exercises, as described in Part 6. These five simple exercises, when done daily, are quite effective at keeping your hormonal system in balance.

Skin-spiration

The Fountain of Youth exercises (see Chapter 24) are so powerful at balancing hormonal levels that some women may start having menstrual cycles again. Don't be concerned. Welcome them. Your body is responding healthily. And don't be concerned if your menstrual cycles don't return. Everyone's body is different.

♦ Use progesterone cream to help keep your hormones in balance. Progesterone cream is available without a prescription at health food stores and pharmacies. Use exactly as directed on the label. After several months, you may be able to reduce the amount and still get great benefit. Discuss this option with your health care provider.

♦ Eat foods containing *phytoestrogens*, which act like estrogen in the body when eaten. They can soothe menopausal discomfort and support the hormonal levels of all the body's many hormones. These foods include figs, dates, pomegranates, fennel, apricots, flax seeds, apples, sprouts, peas, parsley, and raspberries.

♦ Some herbs also contain phytoestrogens. They include black cohosh, chasteberry, red clover, licorice, raspberry leaf, and ginseng. Use herbs as tinctures or tea. Use sparingly, as they can produce strong results.

♦ Take nutritional supplements made from wild yam that contain *dioscorea*. This aids you body in producing hormones.

♦ Maintain an active sex life. You'll be healthier overall. Sex stimulates the production of reproductive hormones. If your sex drive has waned with the onset of menopause, ask your doctor about testosterone and its possible benefits.

By taking positive action on these suggestions, you can keep your body healthy and radiant through menopause and beyond. Everything you do will benefit your skin.

Clarifying Words _____

Phytoestrogens are estrogen-like compounds found in foods. When you eat these foods, they act like the estrogens produced in the body. Phytoestrogens are weaker than the estrogen your body produces. Estrogen helps keep your skin thicker with higher levels of elastin and collagen. **Dioscorea** is a nutrient contained in wild yam. It's not a phytoestrogen, but serves as a precursor to progesterone. The body can produce progesterone and other hormones from dioscorea.

Skin Care for Menopause

Now that you've begun to take care of your body so that your energy and vitality are high, it's time to discuss skin treatments. Here's what to do.

- ◆ Continue your daily skin ritual of cleansing, toning, and moisturizing. If your skin is too dry, you may need to switch skin care products. Do some research and find a skin care line that is formulated to work for menopausal and post-menopausal skin.

- ◆ Continue to exfoliate regularly to remove dead skin cells from the surface of your skin. Use a very gentle exfoliant, as your skin may now be more sensitive to stronger scrubs and acids.

- ◆ To correct any skin discoloration caused by the slowing down of melanin production, use skin lighteners, either as cosmeceuticals or by prescription, such as hydroquinone.

- ◆ Continue your daily sunscreen application. This protects skin from sun damage as well as helps to avoid skin pigmentation discoloration.

- ◆ Have your skin checked regularly by your health care provider for skin cancers and have any removed.

- ◆ Use skin care products and treatments containing cosmeceuticals that help reverse the signs of aging. Such ingredients could include alpha lipoic acid, antioxidants, DMAE, bioflavinoids, and vitamin C.

Be gentle and forgiving with your skin. Because your skin has changed, it may take some time for you to understand its needs and how to care for it.

CAUTION

Wrinkle Guard _____

Many soy products are touted as excellent sources of phytoestrogens for menopausal women. Soybeans in their natural state, such as green edamame, are beneficial. But be careful about eating concentrated soy products, such as soy protein, more often than once or twice a week. They contain concentrated amounts of phytoestrogens. If you enjoy tofu and tempeh, eat them occasionally, but avoid eating them more than once or twice a week. Frequent ingestion of soy products has been shown to produce undesirable side effects such as thyroid disorders and dementia in some people.

Serious Medical Repair

You may be considering plastic surgery or other medical procedures such as laser resurfacing to bring back a youthful appearance to your skin and face.

Bravo. We're all for it. We cover these procedures in detail in Part 7 of this book.

Once you have made the decision to go ahead with a procedure, be sure to do your research. Find several board-certified surgeons with excellent credentials who can advise you concerning what corrections can be made and what you can realistically expect. Interview the surgeons until you find one with whom you can communicate well. Ask for recommendations from friends, your doctor, and other health care practitioners.

Don't expect miracles. That's not the purpose of plastic surgery. What you can expect is to look fresher and more relaxed. The sags and bags will be gone, your skin won't be as loose, and you'll appear 10 to 15 years younger.

Plastic surgery doesn't keep you from aging any further. It just turns back the clock a bit. Most people who have plastic surgery find they want another procedure done in about 10 years.

Your lifestyle makes a big difference in the ultimate success of any surgery. Be sure to maintain your menopausal health, fitness, and diet plan, and you'll look your best.

Male Menopause

Scientists aren't quite sure if men go through a hormonally induced change in middle age, but men certainly change. These changes are just not as drastic or clear as those in women.

For instance, we know that men's bodies produce testosterone throughout their lives, which is why men can father children well into their 80s or 90s, provided their partner is young enough to conceive. But in middle age men's bodies change. They gain weight in their midsections. Their hair changes—it gets gray and thins and some men lose all of their hair.

Men can stay with their daily skin care ritual for life unless their skin begins to feel too dry. If so, switch to products that give your skin more moisture. Continue to exfoliate regularly. Use skin lighteners if you have deeper pigmentation in some areas of your face. Apply sunscreen every morning and more often if you are outdoors in the sun.

Men's skin doesn't droop and sag like women's from a change of life. But men can still have drooping and sagging from sun damage and unhealthy lifestyles. Change your lifestyle and use sun protection to help your skin rejuvenate. Plastic surgery is a viable option for men as well as women.

The Least You Need to Know

- Menopause causes significant changes to skin that make it appear older and aged.

- Menopausal skin can appear radiant and refreshed with a healthy lifestyle and proper skin care treatments.

- Use phytoestrogen-containing foods to boost estrogen levels in the body and mitigate some menopausal skin concerns.

- Men experience skin aging without the drastic changes that women experience.

20

Skin Loves Water

In This Chapter

- ◆ Water: The body's essential ingredient
- ◆ Keeping skin hydrated from the inside out
- ◆ How to drink water
- ◆ Balancing electrolytes

Each and every one of your trillions of skin cells needs water. In fact, every cell of your body needs water. Water is the most essential nutrient for your body. It's required for every bodily and metabolic function occurring within you.

Human beings can survive for about five weeks without eating food. But if a person tried to go without water for only three to five days, he or she couldn't survive. Water is that important. Water keeps you alive. It also keeps your skin healthy and beautiful. Don't underestimate the power of this important nutrient.

In this chapter, you'll learn all about why drinking about eight glasses or more of purified water every day is essential to having perfect skin. You'll discover exactly how much water your body requires based on your body weight, what kind of water to drink, and how to develop a taste for plain old H_2O.

Thirsting for Water

A large percentage of your body is made up of water. The amount of water in a man who is at his ideal size is 60 to 65 percent. That's almost two-thirds of his body. A woman at her ideal size has a water content of between 55 and 60 percent. These amounts are considered to be ideal hydration levels.

A person who is overweight has a lower percentage of water in his or her body. The increase in body fat that comes with being overweight reduces the amount of hydration in the body. People who are overweight are constantly dehydrated, at water percentages of 50 percent or lower, making it harder to lose the excess pounds. That's why dieters are frequently reminded to drink plenty of water—it helps the body release fat.

Skin-spiration

When your skin feels dry, by all means apply more moisturizer, but also drink a glass or two of purified water at the same time. Drinking plenty of water makes your whole body and your skin work well. Dry skin is caused by genetics, environment, illness, and aging. Be sure to read Chapter 14 to learn how to correct dehydrated skin.

When your body becomes even slightly dehydrated, as in a drop of less than one percent below normal levels, you have a decline in blood volume. This in turn triggers the hypothalamus—the brain's thirst center—to make you thirsty by increasing the sodium levels in your blood.

Wrinkle Guard

When you are dehydrated, your metabolic rate slows down. This means that your skin functions also slow down. Skin cell turnover rate decreases, sebum production decreases, and even the healing rate of breakouts decreases. The bottom line is: Drink plenty of water.

When you get thirsty, be sure to drink more than enough water to quench your thirst. Drinking only enough water to relieve the symptom of thirst can actually keep you dehydrated.

With age, a person's sense of thirst becomes dulled, at the very time when skin naturally becomes drier. So be sure to drink at least eight glasses of water every day even if you don't feel thirsty.

Dehydration and Your Skin

Water is the fluid of life. When you don't drink enough water, the dehydration shows up on your skin in more ways than just surface dryness. Without an adequate amount of water to keep your body properly hydrated, here's what happens to your skin.

- Waste products from within the skin can't be flushed efficiently, leaving the skin looking dull and dingy.

- Your digestive system needs water to convert food into fuel. When dehydrated, the digestive waste products may seek exit through the skin, causing eruptions and breakouts.

- Normal elimination can slow down and toxins build up in the large intestine and colon, resulting in skin eruptions.

- Skin cell turnover slows, making skin unresponsive to treatments.

- Perimenopausal and menopausal "hot flashes" can often exacerbate rosacea and other skin eruptions. Drinking a full glass of water can ease hot flashes.

- Puffy eyes and baggy eyes can be the result of water retention, which is often caused by inadequate water consumption.

- Edema and swelling of the face and skin can also be caused by inadequate water consumption.

- Dehydration can intensify the symptoms of health disorders, such as diabetes, high blood pressure, mood disorders, and some autoimmune disorders.

- Dehydration causes fatigue, which shows up on your face.

- Dehydration encourages an increase in inflammatory compounds that create skin damage.

The vision of perfect skin—dewy, moist, plump, and radiant—requires water. The good news is that water is readily available, abundant, inexpensive, and easy to consume.

Drinking Your Water

Your body craves water. Every cell wants you to drink water. You can calculate exactly how much water your cells crave by using this simple formula: Take your body weight in pounds. Divide by two. That's the number of ounces of water your body needs on a normal day.

For example, if you weight 150 pounds, you need 75 ounces of water a day. Assuming that an average glass of water contains 8 ounces, you need 9.375 glasses of water. Always round up the number of glasses, so for a person who weighs 150 pounds, he or she needs to drink 10 glasses of water every day.

This chart gives you amount of water per body weight:

120 pounds	8 glasses
150 pounds	10 glasses
175 pounds	11 glasses
200 pounds	13 glasses
250 pounds	16 glasses
300 pounds	19 glasses

Consider that amount of water to be your bottom line—the lowest amount you'll consume daily. But what about days that aren't normal, such as …

◆ Days when you exercise vigorously, hopefully at least three days a week?

◆ Days spent out-of-doors?

◆ Hot days in the middle of the summer or on vacation?

◆ Living in a climate with low humidity, such as the southwestern United States?

◆ Living in freezing climates with very low humidity in the winter, such as Minnesota or Alaska?

◆ Airline travel (pressurized cabins with extremely low humidity are dehydrating)?

◆ Drinking alcoholic beverages that dehydrate you?

◆ Drinking caffeinated beverages, such as coffee, tea, diet sodas, and regular sodas?

Skin-spiration

Many liquids, such as alcoholic beverages, sodas, diet sodas, coffee, tea, and juice, can be harmful to the quality of your skin because they cause a rapid rise in blood sugar levels which leads to inflammation.

When any or all of these conditions are present, you need to drink more water than your minimum. From a technical point of view, any liquid you consume can contribute to hydrating your body. But we aren't just talking about getting enough liquid, we are discussing having great skin. And your skin performs best when you drink purified water, not just any old liquid.

Drinking fluids is not the same thing as drinking water. Many fluids are actually dehydrating to your body, such as alcoholic and caffeinated beverages. If you consume these, you may need to drink even more water to compensate for their dehydrating effects.

A Refreshing Break

Go ahead. Take a water break. Or sip on your water throughout the day. Either way, you'll be giving your skin a treatment.

What you don't want to do is drink all of your daily water allotment at one time. That would actually be detrimental and, quite honestly, useless. You can overdose on water. If a person drinks too much water all at once, the body's equilibrium gets unbalanced. Too much water isn't a skin treatment, it's skin and body damage.

If you get too busy during the day to pay attention to your water consumption, try this. Set a filled gallon water pitcher at your work area. Make sure that, by the end of the day, you have polished off the water and the pitcher is empty.

Don't count on thirst to guide you in drinking enough water. When you are really busy, it's easy to ignore hunger and thus forget to eat. It's even easier to ignore thirst.

Bring along a water bottle when you travel, when you go shopping, and even when you go to the movies or the theater. Have plenty of water on hand for exercise sessions and outdoor activities.

Skin-spiration

Don't be concerned about needing to run to the bathroom every hour or so when you are drinking your minimum allotment of water each day. It's actually better for your body to get up and move around every hour anyway.

The Nontaste of Water

Some people claim to dislike the taste of water. They claim it doesn't taste like anything. Actually, it's not supposed to. The taste of water should be bland and totally unexciting. Because water makes up large portion of your body, the taste of purified water should be in harmony with you and undistinguishable.

If you are accustomed to always consuming fluids that have flavor, starting out with plain water may seem unsatisfying. Unfortunately, there's absolutely nothing to add to water to give it flavor that doesn't change the water into something else. Even a squeeze of lemon turns the water acidic.

Give the plain and boring taste of purified water a try. Remember, drinking purified water is a skin treatment. It doesn't necessarily need to be exciting or delicious. It only needs to be good for your skin.

Purified Water

The quality of our water supply is in the news frequently. Experts are concerned about the pollutants and chemicals in tap water. Government officials vote on the allowable tolerances for poisonous substances such as arsenic in our drinking supply.

The best solution to avoid potential health risks is not to drink tap water. Instead, drink purified water as often as possible. Here are some good sources for purified water:

◆ Install a water purifier for the whole house or put one under the kitchen sink. Choose from reverse osmosis systems, carbon filtration systems, and distillation. Do your research before you purchase, taking into consideration the annual cost of filters, cost of installation, and overall purity of the water.

◆ Have purified bottled water delivered weekly to your home or office.

◆ Purchase bottled water as needed. It can be expensive if you do this every day, but it's great for special events and situations. You don't need to drink the fancy—and expensive—bottled waters. Some feature carbonation, special minerals, or alkaline formulations. If you enjoy them, go ahead and drink them, but for the purpose of great skin, regular purified water works best.

Clarifying Words

Electrolytes are mineral salts that, in solution, conduct a current of electricity. Electrolytes are required by cells to regulate the flow of water molecules across cell membranes. Major electrolytes are sodium, potassium, chloride, calcium, magnesium, bicarbonate, phosphate, and sulfate.

Electrolyte Balancing

If you're drinking plenty of water, yet still feel dehydrated, it could be that your *electrolytes* are out of balance. Lack of adequate electrolytes in the body results in feelings of fatigue, exhaustion, and intensified stress levels.

Your electrolytes get out of balance through sweating, exercise, poor nutrition, stress, and illness. They can also get out of balance from regular living. When your electrolytes are low or out of balance, your body can't make use of the water you drink, so the water is excreted without hydrating your body.

Replenish electrolytes through eating balanced meals. You can also replenish by using electrolyte replenishment drinks. The best is Emergen-C. It comes in small, one-serving packets. When the contents are mixed into a glass of water, it forms over 32 mineral complexes of electrolytes. Plus, Emergen-C includes B vitamins for replenishment. Emergen-C tastes good, is sweetened with fructose, and only contains 20 calories. It's also available in a wide assortment of flavors, such as tropical, orange, lemon-lime, and cranberry. You can purchase it at your health food store. Some grocery stores carry Emergen-C with the health food products.

Some people drink Gatorade or other sugared electrolyte drinks for electrolyte replenishment. We don't recommend these, as they contain sugars that raise blood glucose levels, plus artificial colorings and flavors, none of which are good for your skin. These ingredients cause inflammation and actually detract from the appearance of your skin.

You can rebalance your electrolytes by taking electrolyte supplements available at the health food store. Be sure to drink the recommended amount of water when using them.

Humidity

If you live in a humid climate, it's easier to have great skin. The moisture in the air helps keep your skin dewy and moist. You lose less moisture from your skin on a day-to-day basis than people who live in dry climates. In dry climates, water evaporates from the surface of your skin into the atmosphere. Your skin feels drier and you need to use skin care products that draw moisture to the surface of your skin. You may even need a heavier moisturizer for the daytime.

If you live in a dry climate, consider using a humidifier to add moisture back into the air. Your best bet is one that attaches to your furnace and air conditioner. It continually adds moisture. If this is unfeasible, or if you work in an office environment, consider using a portable room humidifier. Your skin will radiate its appreciation.

Too Much Water

Although adequate amounts of water are good for you, too much water can be bad for you. If you drink too much water at one time, you'll make yourself sick. If you expose your skin to too much water, you could harm it. Too much water exposure on hands and other areas of the body can result in contact dermatitis. This makes the skin red, irritated, and itchy.

CAUTION

Wrinkle Guard

Hot tubs can be soothing to your psyche but bad for your skin and health. Bacteria can grow rapidly in hot tubs that are poorly maintained. The bacteria causes skin rashes and respiratory diseases. It's estimated that over half of the hot tubs at spas, health clubs, and hotels are poorly maintained.

Prolonged water exposure disrupts the protective surface of the skin. Be sure to thoroughly dry your hands after washing and apply a protective hand cream. Avoid immersing your skin in water for longer than 10 to 15 minutes at a time. Limit your time in the hot tub, bathtub, swimming pool, ocean, or lake.

Steam can be great for your skin when used by a professional skin care technician during a facial. But too much steam, as in a steam room, can actually cause dehydration and inflammation. Go easy on the steam.

The Least You Need to Know

◆ Drink eight or more glasses of purified water every day.

◆ Your skin needs water for cell replenishment, detoxification, and to stay plump and moist.

◆ Drinking other fluids, such as sodas and coffee, doesn't give you the same benefits as drinking purified water.

◆ Use electrolyte nutritional supplements to help your body stay hydrated.

Chapter 21

Feeding Your Skin

In This Chapter

- Balancing your food intake
- Eating proteins, fats, and carbohydrates
- Eating low-glycemic carbs
- Adding nutritional supplements

Puffy donuts, french fries, and mashed potatoes are renowned as all-time favorite comfort foods. While they may comfort you when tired or anxious, they sure don't comfort your skin. Anything but. They deplete your skin's radiance and vibrancy. But you probably already knew that.

What you may not know is what to eat to enhance your skin's glow and beauty. Every time you eat, you are nourishing your skin with health-filled foods or you are depleting its energy with inflammation-creating foods.

Fortunately, *nutrient-dense* foods that benefit your skin are also delicious, energizing, and fun to eat. In this chapter, you'll learn about the foods that beautify your skin from the inside out. You'll also learn which foods to eat sparingly, if at all, and which foods to avoid entirely.

Clarifying Words _____

Nutrient-dense foods contain more vitamins, minerals, and antioxidants plus more complete protein, good fats, and good carbs than other foods. These nutrients benefit the appearance of your skin. An avocado is a nutrient-dense food, as is a carrot. Donuts and french fries aren't.

Nutrition at a Glance

Your skin and body want the best nutrition all the time. They don't react well to foods devoid of vitamins, minerals, and antioxidants. If your skin could talk, it undoubtedly would tell you what foods make it feel good and which ones don't.

In a very real sense, though, your skin does talk to you. Not with words, but certainly through its behavior. Redness, inflammation, breakouts, dry skin, and many other undesirable skin conditions can result from poor nutrition.

You may be confused as you read diet books and articles about nutrition as to what is good nutrition and what is poor nutrition. In this section, you'll learn the simple basics.

Essentially, there are only four kinds of foods you can eat. They are proteins, carbohydrates, fats, and artificial foods. Your body requires the first three—proteins, carbohydrates, and fats. For the best nutrition, eat these in a balanced way, not excluding any of them. Your body has absolutely no need for artificial foods, however. Artificial foods, which are created in the laboratory, are present in most processed foods.

Artificial foods include artificial sweeteners, trans fatty acids, partially hydrogenated vegetable oils, artificial colorings, monosodium glutamate, and most food preservatives. If you can't pronounce the ingredient, most likely, it's an artificial food.

Proteins

At every meal, your body needs protein that contains all nine essential amino acids. Protein substances form your muscles, ligaments, tendons, organs, glands, nails, hair, and skin. Skin contains the proteins collagen and elastin.

Without adequate protein, your skin ages prematurely and loses elasticity and firmness. The skin becomes dull and artificially pale, the muscles in the face lose strength, and—in severe cases of protein deprivation—hair falls out and nails weaken and split.

The only food source of *complete protein* is animal products, such as meats, fish, poultry, seafood, and eggs. Cheese contains complete protein, but may not be your best choice, as you'll see later when we discuss balanced eating.

An average-sized woman requires about 20 grams of animal protein three times a day, or 60 grams a day. Twenty grams is about the size of a deck of cards, or a small can of tuna fish. No, you don't need to eat a 16-ounce rib-eye steak every evening to obtain adequate protein. In fact, that steak could feed four people the amount of protein they need for one meal.

Clarifying Words

Complete protein designates a food that contains all nine essential amino acids. Only animal-based foods contain complete proteins.

Men require more protein, up to about 30 grams of protein three times a day—or about one-and-a-half small cans of tuna.

Eating all of your daily allotment of protein in one meal isn't a good idea. That much protein taxes your digestive, assimilation, and elimination systems. Your body functions best when you feed it smaller amounts of complete protein throughout the day. That way, your energy levels are stabilized and you can avoid late afternoon fatigue. Eat complete protein for breakfast, lunch, and dinner. You can even include a serving of protein with your snacks.

Wrinkle Guard

Some vegetarians recommend using food combining as a way to ingest all nine amino acids at a meal without eating animal products, such as by combining legumes with rice, corn, nuts, seeds, or wheat. Unfortunately for the condition of your skin, eating the high load of starchy carbohydrates that food combining requires causes skin inflammation. Inflammation is caused by eating too much sugar and too much starch because they trigger hyperinsulinism and insulin resistance. Vegetarians can counteract this by eating fish, cheese, or eggs at every meal and cutting back on starches and sugars.

Fats

If you've been eating a low-fat diet, now's the time to give it up for good. Eating low fat doesn't work long-term for weight loss. Depriving your body of fat deprives your skin of cherished nutrients. The American Heart Association recommends a diet with 30 percent fat in your daily food intake. You don't need to restrict your fat to percentages lower than that.

Of all the fats available at the grocery store, you only need three for health:

◆ Essential fatty acids (EFAs)

◆ Olive oil

◆ Butter

Essential Fatty Acids (EFAs)

These are so important to the health of your skin and your entire being that we recommend you take these as food supplements as well as eat foods containing them, such as salmon and sardines. Essential fatty acids make your skin glow. They reduce inflammation, and are beneficial for any skin condition, from dehydration to premature aging. They improve the conditions of eczema and psoriasis. They aid in the transmission of nerve impulses and assist your brain neurotransmitters in working correctly. They ease mood disorders, such as depression and anxiety. Plus, they've been shown to reduce insulin resistance, which can lead to diabetes.

Essential fatty acids are known as Omega-6 and Omega-3 acids. Omega-6 EFAs help restore parts of the epidermis, while Omega-3 EFAs restore collagen and elastin.

You can purchase EFAs at the grocery store or health food store. Look for fish oil capsules, cod liver oil, or salmon oil capsules. These animal-based EFAs are important for your skin because they contain docosahexaenoic (DHA) and eicosapentaenoic (EPA) Omega-3 acids. Vegetable-based EFAs, such as flax seeds, are missing these acids. However, the vegetable EFAs like flax seed oil, borage oil, and evening primrose oil do contain alpha linolenic acids and other Omega-6 EFAs that benefit your health and skin.

> **Wrinkle Guard**
>
> Avoid eating farmed salmon, as it contains harmful growth chemicals and colorings. At present, albacore tuna contains high levels of mercury. Instead, eat other kinds of tuna. As best we know, they don't contain undesirable pollutants. You can also order fresh wild salmon online.

Take 2 tablespoons of essential fatty acids daily, or the equivalent in fish oil capsules. In addition, eat wild salmon or sardines at least twice a week (canned salmon and sardines are wild). More is better. As a boost, you can also grind up flax seeds to sprinkle on salads and vegetables.

Olive Oil

This is your best choice for salads and dressing vegetables. Olive oil is *cold-expeller pressed* from olives. It's fresh and good for you. Other vegetable oils are usually processed with heat. When this happens, the oils become partially hydrogenated, and that's a problem. Partially hydrogenated vegetable oils are also known as trans-fatty acids. Trans-fatty acids directly cause heart disease. Avoid eating them.

If you can find cold-expeller pressed vegetable oils, such as canola oil, walnut oil, and peanut oil, you can use them for salads and dressing vegetables as well. The best olive oil is first pressed and comes from areas of Spain and the Mediterranean. It contains the highest levels of antioxidants, which are great for your skin.

Don't heat olive oil or vegetable oils, because when you do, they become partially hydrogenated and can harm your health. If you want to be totally on the safe side, don't even sauté vegetables in olive oil. You are making yourself a concoction of trans-fatty acids. The same goes for using oils for baking. Use butter instead.

Clarifying Words

Cold-expeller pressed oils are oils that are extracted from the vegetables without heat. Most other vegetables oils available in the grocery stores, such as canola and corn oils, are heat extracted. Purchase only cold-expeller pressed vegetable oils because they don't contain trans-fatty acids.

Avoid eating all processed foods that contain partially hydrogenated vegetable oils, because they are a direct ticket to heart disease. And they certainly aren't good for your skin.

The Food and Drug Administration requires that by January 1, 2006, all food manufacturers list trans-fatty acids on their nutrition labels. The FDA estimates that by January 1, 2009, trans-fat labeling will prevent anywhere from 600 to 1,200 cases of coronary heart disease and 250 to 500 deaths each year.

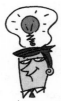

Skin-spiration

One of the best things you can do for your skin through nutrition is to toss out any low-fat food you have in your kitchen. Toss out low-fat mayonnaise, low-fat salad dressings, and fake butter. Toss out margarine, vegetable-based frying fat, and any processed foods labeled "low-fat." They are filled with the artificial ingredients that cause inflammation and they usually contain high-glycemic ingredients.

Butter

This is an excellent fat for baking and heating. It doesn't decompose into trans-fatty acids and it tastes great. In small amounts, it's perfectly healthy for you and good for your skin.

Avoid using large amounts of butter because it's a saturated fat. The American Heart Association recommends eating only 10 percent of your food intake in saturated fats.

Keep these three types of fat handy in your kitchen. You'll have all the fats you need for cooking, baking, eating, and for maintaining healthy and radiant skin.

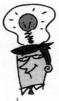

> **Skin-spiration**
>
> As you read through this list of fats beneficial for your skin, you may be wondering what oils to use for frying food, such as chicken and French fries. Most likely, you won't be frying food. You don't need to. Frying with oils is really bad for your skin because of the high concentration of trans-fatty acids. The hotter the oil, the higher the concentration of trans-fatty acids. Again, avoid them for better skin.

Carbohydrates

For healthy skin, you need plenty of carbohydrates in your daily food intake. Yes, that's right, carbohydrates. If you are familiar with low-carb diets, you may think of carbohydrates as bad for you. That's not exactly accurate. What's bad for you are too many of the wrong kinds of carbohydrates.

Plenty of the good carbohydrates are great for your skin. The type of carbohydrate you eat makes all the difference in the health and beauty of your skin.

There are four kinds of carbohydrates:

- ◆ Starches. Includes grains, breads, muffins, cookies, cakes, donuts, pasta, and bagels. Rice, millet, oatmeal, flour, and breakfast cereals are all starches. The base of pizza is a starch, as are tortillas. White potatoes behave in the body as starch, so they fit into the starch category. Corn is also in this category.

- ◆ Sugars. Includes table sugar, honey, high-fructose corn syrup, and molasses.

- ◆ Fruits. Includes all natural fruits, such as apples, oranges, melons, berries, papaya, kiwi, pears, and many more.

- ◆ Vegetables. Includes all the green vegetables, such as lettuce, kale, green beans, broccoli, and peas. Add in cauliflower, fennel, tomatoes, cucumbers, radishes, sweet potatoes, and carrots. The types of vegetables are endless.

The best carbohydrates to eat are the vegetables and fruits, the ones to avoid are the starches, and the ones to eat sparingly are the sugars, with the exception of high-fructose corn syrup.

The reason to avoid starches is that they create inflammation. Here's how.

Whenever you eat a carbohydrate, your blood sugar level rises, sometimes slightly and sometimes dramatically, depending on the type of carbohydrate. In general, starches trigger a higher and faster rise. Vegetables hardly affect blood sugar levels at all.

The higher and faster your blood sugar level rises, the more insulin your pancreas excretes. The insulin reduces the level of sugar, also known as glucose, in your blood. So far, this is healthy. But when your blood sugar rises frequently because your diet is high in starches, the continual rise in blood sugar causes inflammation in the blood vessels and the cells, and ultimately, in your skin.

When your pancreas is producing large amounts of insulin often, your body becomes insulin-resistant, meaning it requires more and more insulin to reduce blood sugar levels. The result for your skin: more inflammation. The result for your body: weight gain, increase in LDL (bad) cholesterol levels, fatigue, and higher susceptibility to adult-onset diabetes.

This entire cycle of a swift rise in blood sugar and insulin overproduction creates stress in the body and increases cortisol levels. That level of stress isn't good for your skin.

Researchers at the University of Sydney in Australia have quantified the effect of certain carbohydrates on blood sugar levels. They measured the increase in blood sugar levels for hundreds of carbohydrates. Their result is the glycemic index.

The glycemic index ranks carbohydrates as high glycemic (70 or higher), medium glycemic (56–60), and low glycemic (55 or less). To learn more about the glycemic index, visit www.mendosa.com.

This list gives you an idea of which foods are high, medium, and low glycemic:

- High-glycemic foods are white and whole wheat bread, rice cakes, pastries, cakes, white potatoes, and cookies. Avoid eating these. Eating these foods indirectly causes a rise in cortisol levels, so these foods trigger the release of cortisol, a stress hormone. Eating these foods can make you feel more stressed. We'll talk more about cortisol inducers in Chapter 22. They also cause inflammation in the body and skin.

- Medium-glycemic foods are table sugar, honey, and molasses. Dark chocolate and some combined foods, such as lemon mousse, are medium glycemic. Eat these sparingly.

- Low-glycemic foods are vegetables and most fruits. Eat plenty of these. You need 5 to 10 servings every day.

Modifying your diet according to the glycemic index is a great start, but as people began to use the glycemic index, some found that their blood sugar levels were rising to high levels in spite of eating low-glycemic foods. Why? Because they were eating too much of a good thing. In other words, one apple is great, five apples at one sitting equals trouble.

Enter the concept of glycemic load value. This calculation lets you know the quantity of a food that will give you good results—or bad ones. It's suggested that a person's glycemic load count for a whole day be between 130 and 160. Persons with diabetes need to eat under 100 daily.

You can find a complete glycemic listing of all carbohydrates, including glycemic load, at www.mendosa.com. You can also purchase an inexpensive computer program called GlycoLoad, available to download for $15.95 at www.phelpsteam.com/glycoload. This program calculates glycemic load based on grams as well as ounces, which is great for those of us living in the United States.

Now, let's get practical. Starches are a mainstay of our national diet. How does a person avoid them when they seem to be everywhere? When you order in pizza, include a salad with your order. Eat the top of a couple slices of pizza, toss out the bread and eat the salad. When you order a hamburger, toss out the bun and eat the meat. Add a side salad.

Eating without starches takes some getting used to. But your skin and your body will thank you.

Artificial Foods

To say the least, artificial foods are controversial. They include artificial sweeteners, chemical preservatives, food colorings, and artificial fats.

While no food manufacturer says they are actually good for you, they claim that they're harmless. Few of these substances have stood the test of time, primarily because most of them haven't been in the food supply long enough.

Until artificial foods have been used and tested on thousands of people for about 25 years, we have no way of knowing whether they are truly safe. Until such a time arrives, avoid eating artificial foods. We certainly know that they aren't good for your skin.

Eating in Harmony with Your DNA

Now that you understand the kinds of foods you can eat for healthy skin, let's set them into a framework so you can understand how the different kinds of foods work in your body.

Some foods are totally compatible with your DNA. Other foods aren't. We know from scientific research that our present-day DNA is virtually identical to that of the caveman and cavewoman's. Over seven million years, the foods they ate became compatible with their DNA, which is our DNA today. These foods are called Paleo foods. Here's what the caveman and cavewoman ate:

◆ Animal proteins, such as meat, fish, and poultry

◆ Nuts and seeds

◆ Vegetables and fruits, including edamame (fresh green soy beans) and berries

◆ Eggs

◆ Honey

◆ Herbs and spices

You can eat and digest these foods with ease. Few people are allergic to whole categories of these foods (even if your children would like you to believe they're allergic to vegetables). These foods are low glycemic. These foods are good for your skin. You could possibly be allergic to one of these foods. If so, don't eat it.

A second category of foods is called Neo foods. Humans have eaten them for only 10,000 years or less. These foods haven't been in the food chain long enough for human DNA to adapt well to them. Humans began eating these foods after the domestication of animals, which took place about 10,000 years ago. These foods include:

◆ Dairy, cheese, milk, ice cream

◆ Grains, breads, flour, rice

◆ White potatoes and corn as we know them today

Skin-spiration

Herbs and spices boost your skin's health. They are filled with antioxidants and health-giving nutrients. Use them to enhance the taste of all your meals and your skin will benefit as well.

Wrinkle Guard

Don't turn up your nose at those stinky vegetables—cabbage, broccoli, brussels sprouts, and cauliflower. These cruciferous vegetables are excellent for your skin health. Eat them frequently.

Wrinkle Guard

If you're hooked on soy shakes for breakfast, keep the shake, but lose the soy. Instead, add whey powder to your shake. That way you're getting all nine essential amino acids, without the worries of eating too much soy, which can lead to serious problems like thyroid disorders and dementia. If you want to eat Paleo foods, consider eggs with fruit for breakfast.

Skin-spiration

If you have a skin autoimmune disorder, such as psoriasis, eczema, seborrhea, or rosacea, eliminate Neo foods from your diet for one month. If your condition improves, continue eating Paleo foods.

- Soy protein isolate as contained in soy shakes and protein bars
- Chocolate
- Coffee
- Alcoholic beverages
- Artificial foods

Plenty of people are allergic to whole categories of these foods, such as dairy or wheat. They are high glycemic or medium glycemic. People with autoimmune disorders who stop eating these foods often regain their health.

Ideally, for both your skin and your overall health, you would eat Paleo foods exclusively, because they're totally compatible with your DNA. But realistically, people love baked goods and ice cream. So here's how to have a bit of your cake and eat it too: Eat Paleo foods for about 80 to 85 percent of your daily intake and eat Neo foods less often, around 15 to 20 percent of your daily food intake.

Make adjustments to those ratios if you aren't getting great results with your skin and health.

Supplementation

Even the best food plan can use a little help. If you eat only the best foods, your body may not be able to completely digest and assimilate all the nutrients you need. That's why supplementation in the form of nutritional supplements is so vital to the beauty of your skin.

Here are some recommendations:

- Essential fatty acids, as discussed earlier in this chapter in the section "Fats."

- B-vitamin complex, either in capsule or liquid form. Often the liquid Bs are more easily assimilated in the body.

- Digestive enzymes. Digestion slows with age, and by the mid-30s a person may not be digesting completely. Take digestive enzymes that include ingredients for digestion of protein, carbohydrates, and fats. Ask the sales consultant at the health food store for recommendations. Take with meals only.

◆ Trace elements. Purchase a formulation that contains over 72 minerals. Anything less than that and you'll be missing something important. Great for reducing stress and keeping skin looking vibrant.

◆ Greens drinks. Contain plenty of antioxidants for skin health. Keep the body slightly alkaline, which can aid with skin conditions such as eczema, psoriasis, seborrhea, and rosacea. Reduce yeast overgrowth syndrome that can result in skin rashes.

◆ Emergen-C for electrolyte, vitamin, and mineral replenishment. Use for fatigue and after exercise. At parties, ask for a glass of mineral water. Add the contents of a pack of Emergen-C and you'll enjoy a truly healthy cocktail (and your eyes won't be swollen in the morning).

You can include other supplements, such as acidophilus, the good intestinal bacteria and specific antioxidants, if they work well for you and your body.

The Least You Need to Know

◆ Eating balanced meals of complete protein, good fats, and low-glycemic carbohydrates is great for your skin.

◆ Use the glycemic index and glycemic load information to eat a diet that is noninflammatory.

◆ Take essential fatty acids daily and eat a diet high in cold-water fish, such as salmon and sardines.

◆ Eat foods that are compatible with your DNA.

22

A Skin-Nurturing Environment

In This Chapter

- ◆ Avoiding environmental stressors
- ◆ Controlling cortisol levels
- ◆ Daily stress soothers
- ◆ Avoiding destructive peer pressure

It's amazing how your skin can tell the difference between living in a healthy and loving environment and living a chaotic existence. In a healthy environment, your skin grows more beautiful day by day. With chaos, your skin reacts unhappily to every stress and pollutant.

When your skin thrives, so does the health of your whole body, and vice versa. Therein lies your challenge. In order to have great skin, you must live healthily. That presents a challenge to most people, because the opportunity to live an unbalanced life is everywhere and requires no effort. To live a healthy lifestyle takes discipline, desire, and work. It also takes love.

In this chapter, you'll learn how to create a skin-friendly environment in your home and office, and within yourself.

Stress Is in the Air

Everything in your environment affects your skin—either positively or destructively. This is because environmental conditions cause certain stress responses in your body. For example, loud music, especially if you don't enjoy the music, can put your body into "fight or flight." That may seem obvious to you, but other less obvious situations, such as pollution, sick-building air, and even listening to and viewing negative and violent news can evoke your "fight or flight" response.

CAUTION

Wrinkle Guard _____

Some office buildings and other public buildings have poor air quality. The air conditioning and heating systems are inefficient at filtering out dust and allergens. Many buildings contain fungus and mold growing within the walls and basements. Such buildings are considered to have sick-building syndrome. If you work in such a building, you can protect yourself and your skin by opening a window, if possible. Or purchase a small air purifier and place in near your work area.

Your "fight or flight" response affects your skin. When you are presented with a situation that's stressful, your body begins the stress cycle. Adrenalin excreted by the adrenal glands starts to pump through the body. Adrenaline is known as the "fight or flight" hormone because it gives you plenty of energy—enough to run away from a situation, or enough to stay and fight the battle.

Immediately after your adrenal glands excrete adrenaline, a second hormone, cortisol, is released. Cortisol acts as a master strategist, working to find solutions to handle the situation. Then, when the stressful event comes to a conclusion, the body goes into a recovery phase. The body rests, relaxes, the adrenaline and cortisol dissipate, and life returns to normal.

For example, imagine a caveman being chased by a wooly mammoth. Adrenaline kicks in. His energy levels surge. Cortisol kicks in and the caveman decides to run as fast as he can to the nearest cave, hoping to trick the animal and find safety. He outruns the mammoth, reaching the cave as the animal lumbers on by. Then the caveman recovers his energy in the cave, perhaps takes a nap, relaxes, and gathers his wits about him before he heads for home.

In today's world, our situations have changed. The human "fight or flight" response works exactly the same way, but people seldom have time to recover from the stress and let it dissipate before they enter back into the fray. If you live in a city with air pollution, your only chance to get away from the pollution stress could be your family's annual beach vacation. Even if you don't experience pollution as a stress factor in your life, your body does. If you drive to work, as most of us do, you are in the car driving at least twice a day, often during heavy rush-hour traffic, meaning your stress hormones are surging during your commute.

When the body is continually stressed, cortisol doesn't have a chance to dissipate. It stays active in the body, and you have long-term stress. Cortisol is an interesting hormone. It's great for special stress situations. It's a killer when it stays in the body continuously. Cortisol is at the root of virtually all chronic lifestyle disorders. Elevated cortisol levels can lead to serious disease, such as diabetes, heart disease, autoimmune disease, cancer, high blood pressure, asthma, and more.

Cortisol also causes weight gain around the waist. All by itself, no matter how many calories you eat, cortisol can cause weight gain. And as if that isn't enough, cortisol leads to serious mood disorders, such as depression and anxiety.

Cortisol causes all this damage because it causes inflammation in many areas of the body, including your skin.

All of these health-related concerns can prevent you from having great skin. Inflammation causes damage to collagen and elastin, and it brings on skin eruptions. Inflammation affects skin tone and can create deposits of dark brown pigmentation.

Alas, you no longer live as the caveman did. You live in a busy, stress-filled world. The way to create better skin is twofold:

- Reduce the amount of stress in your environment and your life.
- Take positive actions to decompress and lower your cortisol levels on a daily basis.

First, let's look at what in the environment causes stress and what to do about it.

Skin Stressors

Your body is bombarded with many stressors every day. Some are mild, some more severe, but they all add up to stress and elevated cortisol levels. Here are a few stressors that can harm your skin:

◆ Air pollution. This is a fact of life, but you can plug a simple air purifier into the electrical socket at your home or office. Yes, you can even purchase an air purifier to use in your car. It plugs into the cigarette lighter socket—a much better use for the socket than using it to light up a smoke. Purchase at www.gaiam.com.

◆ Foods you're allergic to and artificial foods. Avoid eating both.

◆ Most tap water. Drink purified water instead.

◆ Breathing odd fumes, such as the fumes of artificial nails, gasoline, paints, etc. If you must use such substances, use only in a well-ventilated area for short periods of time.

◆ Working in factories and other locations filled with pollutants and toxins. If you work at one of these kinds of locations, consider changing locations, or changing your job.

◆ Dust and household dirt. Clean your house frequently. Change litter boxes often.

Wrinkle Guard

Workplace or occupational exposure to pollutants is responsible for over 70,000 deaths and 350,000 cases of illness a year. Those pollutants are bad for your skin, let alone your health.

◆ Sleeping with makeup still on your face. Wash your face before going to bed.

◆ Sleeping with sunscreen or sun block still on your face. Wash your face before going to bed.

◆ Poor air quality. Change air filters in your home every two to three months. This keeps the air fresh and protects your skin from airborne particulates, fungus, bacteria, dust, and allergens.

◆ General workplace conditions. If you work in a place where your skin can pick up dirt and grease, such as in a restaurant kitchen or on a highway repair crew, be sure to thoroughly cleanse your face every night after work. Yes, you should cleanse your face every evening anyway, but if your workplace is particularly conducive to bad skin, you may need to cleanse more thoroughly than usual. Taking workplace conditions into consideration can often heal teenage acne.

◆ New paint, new carpet, new houses, new cars. All of these contain pollutants that create internal stress. When remodeling, be sure to continually air out your home and install an air purifier to reduce airborne toxins.

Practical Skin Considerations

In the midst of taking care of your skin, it can be easy to overlook some of the more obvious environmental do's and don'ts:

♦ Washcloths. Only use fresh clean washcloths. Use once, then launder before using again. Consider doing the same with towels.

♦ Loofahs and skin-washing netting balls (those big puffy net balls). Wash every week in the washing machine with warm or hot water to remove the build up of dead skin cells, fungus, and bacteria.

♦ Pillow cases. Sleep on one side, turn over and sleep on the other side. Launder before using again. Wash bed linens weekly. Buy a new mattress every couple of years.

♦ Daily cleansing cloths. Never reuse a cleansing cloth in an effort to save money. Discard the used cloth after one use. This means you may need to purchase two boxes every month to get 60 washings.

♦ Makeup. Purchase your own skin care products, foundation, and other makeup for eyes, lips, and skin. Use your own and don't share. That way you aren't unknowingly also sharing germs with a friend.

By adopting these simple and practical skin care suggestions, you may find that a skin condition you have clears up within weeks.

CAUTION

Wrinkle Guard

Make sure that your towels and bed linens are completely rinsed of all laundry detergent before using. You may need to put them through a second rinse cycle or use less detergent than the manufacturer recommends. To protect your skin from the additive and bleaches used in laundry detergents, purchase only those labeled, "free." This designation means they don't contain scents or bleaches. You also may also want to avoid using fabric softeners in your dryer as well.

Polluting Thoughts

Negativity creates skin problems. It may sound silly, but, in fact, every time you experience negative emotions, you trigger a whole adrenaline/cortisol response.

Negativity brings with it fear, anxiety, depression, and worry. Cortisol levels increase and the resulting inflammation shows up in your body and on your skin. When your skin is inflamed, it's easy to get even more stressed. A vicious cycle gets started and it's challenging to correct.

Think of it this way: The more you worry about your skin condition, the worse your skin may appear. Simply telling yourself not to worry doesn't help a thing. In fact, it can make things worse. But there's plenty you can do to break the stress-cortisol cycle so that you and your skin can relax and heal.

Correcting Cortisol Overload

You can improve the condition of your skin by regulating your internal levels of cortisol. By taking advantage of recent research on activities that lower cortisol levels, you can take better care of your skin from the inside out.

Scientists and researchers can measure a person's cortisol levels with a saliva test, and they've run studies to determine what activities lower cortisol levels. The results may surprise you.

One hour of yoga substantially lowers cortisol levels. One hour of television has no effect, and chances are that if you spent that hour watching the news, your cortisol levels actually increased. One hour of hanging out on the sofa also has no effect.

Twenty minutes of mediation or contemplative prayer lowers cortisol levels. In other words, the more your entire body and mind relaxes, the more you lower your stress levels. Getting a professional facial or massage also lowers cortisol levels.

Here's a list of what works to reduce cortisol overload:

◆ Getting in water. Take a bath, get in the hot tub, take a shower, or go swimming.

◆ Meditation and contemplative prayer. It doesn't matter if this involves a religious or spiritual focus or not. The mere fact of regularly clearing your mind reduces cortisol levels. Practice meditation once or twice a day.

◆ Yoga or stretching. Do at least 30 minutes two or three times a week.

◆ Personal pamperings, such as facials, massages, manicures, or pedicures.

◆ Massage therapies, such as cranial-sacral or deep-muscle massage.

◆ Vigorous exercise with an aerobic focus.

◆ Body rolling, a deep-massage technique you can do at home. Learn more at www.yamunabodyrolling.com.

◆ Using a back massage roller. In 15 minutes, you'll be very relaxed. Look for the Maxi-Backsie at www.bodytools.com.

◆ Pilates or core-conditioning exercises. Go slow. Focus on the movement. Get strong while you reduce cortisol levels.

◆ Being outside in nature. Garden, go for a hike, or go for a bike ride.

◆ Pursuing a hobby, such as knitting, singing, playing an instrument, or other activities that are calming and soothing.

◆ Journal writing. Sit in a quiet and comforting location and write out your thoughts and feelings.

Skin-spiration

We hope that the cortisol-saliva test will become available for home use soon. It would be wonderful to chart your stress level and to learn what stress-soothing activities benefit you the most.

You get the gist. These activities are relaxing and soothing. They let you take time for yourself without interference from the outside world. Use this list as a way to get started. You may find other stress-soothing techniques that work to lower your stress levels even further.

Take a Sofa Day

If the world is really getting to you and your stress levels seem way too high, take a day off. Don't use the day to get caught up or to run errands. Instead, take the day to lie on the sofa with a really good page-turner of a book, your favorite snacks within reach.

Just enjoy yourself. By the next day, your daily routine will seem easier and more manageable.

Daily Antianxiety Formula

Stress management is just as important as your daily skin care ritual. You cleanse, tone, and wash your face twice a day because your skin requires regular upkeep. Similarly, just by living in the world, you are surrounded by regular environmental stressors, and you need to perform daily stress management.

Do it for your skin to keep it looking beautiful, but the benefits will go far beyond the surface. The results will seem to beautify your very soul, and, of course, lift your moods, keep you fit, and assist in keeping you healthy.

The following is a time-proven stress management formula. It works for everyone and it will work for you. Do the following:

1. Take 2 tablespoons of essential fatty acids every day. You can choose from flax seed oil, a blend of EFAs, fish oil, or fish oil capsules. Fish oil is best. If you use vegetable EFAs, make sure you get at least two to three servings of fish every week. This keeps your skin soft and smooth, moist, dewy, and radiant.

2. Do at least 45 minutes of vigorous aerobic exercise three times a week, or do 20 minutes or more every day. This keeps your metabolism high, keeps your endorphins high, and keeps your mood balanced. It also increases blood flow to the skin, and aids the body in detoxification. You'll learn more about detoxification in Chapter 23.

3. Avoid cortisol-inducing foods and substances. These include alcoholic beverages, caffeine, smoking, and foods you're allergic to. Starches are cortisol inducing. Starches make blood sugar levels rise rapidly, causing a swift increase in insulin production, and ultimately in cortisol production. All cortisol-inducing foods cause inflammation and stressed-out skin.

This formula can look intimidating. Don't be intimidated. Instead, get started and pay attention to how your skin changes within about three months.

Skin-spiration

Following the stress-management formula doesn't mean you'll never eat another cookie ever again. But it does mean that you'll cut way back on starches and other cortisol-inducing foods. You can indulge, but do so wisely. Find out how your body works. Perhaps you can get away with one cookie a week, but a cookie every day could be too much starch for you. Keep observing your skin, your energy levels, and your moods. Make adjustments as needed.

Relationship Stress

Peer pressure, at any age, can be harmful to your skin. A teenager's life is filled with temptations to give in to peer pressure as a way to fit in. Activities such as smoking, drinking alcoholic beverages, and even drinking coffee can harm skin. Add to that hanging out with friends at fast-food restaurants where it's cool to order a shake and fries, and to drink sodas or diet sodas.

There's stress on both sides of this situation—stress to conform and fit in, and stress on the skin when a person does conform. The easiest solution is to avoid anything that leads to lifelong bad habits that harm the skin. Then, avoid the shakes and fries and opt for salad and purified water instead. It sounds sort of boring, but it sure is great for your skin.

Adults also need to review their personal relationships to determine if peer pressure is harming their skin. Such situations could include simple activities like eating cortisol-inducing foods because your partner does, or not taking time for stress soothers every day because a partner is critical or disapproves. The same goes for not washing your face before bed because your partner doesn't.

Ideally, you can reverse the peer pressure and assist your friends or partner in living a healthier lifestyle, but that's not always easy, and it's not necessary. What is important is that you take care of yourself and your skin, regardless of pressure from others and their desires.

The Least You Need to Know

- Manage your environment to reduce stressors that can harm your skin.
- Do stress soothers daily as a way to lower cortisol stress levels.
- Use the antianxiety stress formula daily to manage stress and improve skin radiance.
- When stress levels seem overwhelming, take a day off to relax and replenish your energy.

Chapter 23

Detoxify the Skin by Detoxifying the Body

In This Chapter

- Understanding your toxin load
- Improving skin through body detoxification
- A daily detox plan
- Special detox treatments

Everyone accumulates toxins in the body simply by living and breathing. No matter how healthy your lifestyle, your body will accumulate toxins. They're present in foods, in the air, and in the water we drink.

The presence of toxins in the body affects your skin and how it performs. By undertaking daily detoxification procedures, you can draw some toxins out of your body's cells. We'd like to tell you that all of your toxins can be flushed, but that's generally not the case. However, as you continue to detoxify your body day by day and do your best to avoid ingesting toxins, you can enjoy a healthier body and better-looking skin.

In this chapter, you'll learn methods for detoxifying your body on an ongoing basis so that you can keep your skin performing at optimal levels and keep it looking dewy, moist, and radiant.

The Theory of Detoxification

As you live your life, toxins accumulate. Many more toxins are present in our environment today than 50 or 100 years ago. They seemingly come from everywhere and they manage to find their way into the body's fat cells. All toxins are processed through the liver in order to be eliminated from the body. This is why so many detoxification programs focus on strengthening the liver.

Toxins enter our bodies from air pollution, a wide variety of household-cleaning products, perfumes and bathing products, and even through laundry detergent. They enter our bodies not just through the water we drink, but also from the water we bathe in, from swimming pools, and from hot tubs. Toxins are present in prescription and over-the-counter medications. They even enter the body through application of cosmetics and skin care products. Pesticides are toxins and they enter the body through the foods we eat, as do the steroids and antibiotics used to raise cattle, poultry, and even fish. In a sense, our bodies are all toxic waste dumps.

Toxins are essentially poisons. They can disrupt our hormonal systems, and can be carcinogenic, thus provoking cancer growth. They can exacerbate autoimmune diseases and weaken our body's immune system, making it more susceptible to viral, fungal, and bacterial infections. And, of course, the effects of these toxins show up on the face and skin as congestion, breakouts, and premature aging.

The idea behind detoxification is to assist the body in naturally removing toxins. It would be great if we could simply use a vacuum cleaner and suction out all the toxins, but what works on your living room carpet can't be used within the body. So, in order to detoxify, a person needs to work with the body's systems of organs and glands to help the natural process function properly.

Some detoxification programs that you find in advertisements and at health food stores are used for weight loss, the theory being that fat cells store body toxins, and for a person to lose weight, the fat cells need to release the toxins to be processed by the liver and then eliminated from the body. The detoxification recommendations in this chapter may or may not assist you with weight loss. But they will assist your body in releasing toxins, which will ultimately benefit your skin.

Benefits of Detoxification

You are already aware that your skin mirrors the health and condition of your body. When your body is on toxin overload, it will be revealed in the condition of your skin.

Let's get specific. You can expect certain results from detoxification. Not every person will experience all of these benefits immediately, but over time you can improve the condition of your skin and your health. Here's how you can benefit from a detoxification program:

- ◆ You can reduce skin congestion so that skin is clearer and skin cells turn over faster.

- ◆ You can reduce the frequency of breakouts.

- ◆ You can improve the functioning of your immune system, which can ease autoimmune skin disorders such as psoriasis, eczema, rosacea, and seborrhea.

- ◆ You can alleviate chronic conditions such as yeast overgrowth syndrome and autoimmune diseases.

- ◆ You can improve skin tone.

- ◆ You can reduce skin dryness.

- ◆ You can reduce the signs of premature aging.

- ◆ You can eliminate odd rashes and spots.

The results of a detoxification program are individual. You could experience these results or other, different results depending on your toxin load and your body's healing priorities.

Wrinkle Guard _____

Be careful starting any detoxification plan, because you might feel worse before you feel better. This is sometimes called the cleansing response. As your body flushes out toxins, you could feel irritable, cranky, and—if you are flushing lots of toxins—you could end up with a cold or the flu. So start off by going slow and letting your body and skin take the time they need to release toxins and heal gradually.

Your Daily Detoxification Program

Do the following on a daily basis:

◆ Eat between 20 and 35 grams of fiber a day. When you eat two to three servings of vegetables and fruits at every meal, this is easy. You can also add fiber to your diet as a nutritional supplement. Use psyllium husks, which are widely available at the health food store. Mix 1 teaspoon in a glass of water and drink immediately before it gels. Follow with another glass of purified water. In addition to adding fiber to your diet, the psyllium helps move toxins from the digestive tract so they leave the body through elimination.

◆ Dry brush the body every morning before your shower. The light brushing actually encourages the lymph fluid under the skin to move and carry toxins with it. Purchase a natural bristle brush. These are widely available at discount chains and home-furnishing stores. You can also find natural bristle brushes specifically made for dry brushing at your health food store. Start at your feet, moving up your legs, and lightly brush your skin towards your torso. Then do your arms, brushing towards your heart. Finish up with your neck, chest, back, buttocks, and stomach. You may feel a slight tingling sensation as you brush. This whole process takes only one to two minutes, so you can do this as you wait for the water to get hot in the shower. Dry brushing makes your skin soft and baby smooth. It also gently exfoliates the skin on your body.

> **CAUTION**
>
> **Wrinkle Guard**
>
> Your facial skin is too delicate for dry brushing, so don't dry brush your face, no matter how fine the brush's bristles. Instead, use exfoliation, clay masks, and facials as a way to encourage the lymph fluid under the skin to flush toxins.

◆ Make sure you have a full and complete bowel movement at least once a day. Your natural elimination system works to remove toxins. If you are chronically constipated, check with your doctor for healthful solutions. Eating 5 to 10 servings of vegetables and fruits every day is great for elimination, as is psyllium, mentioned previously. You simply can't detoxify if your bowels aren't eliminating every day.

◆ Do the Fountain of Youth Exercises described in Chapter 24 every day. They only take 5 to 10 minutes and are excellent for detoxifying the body, balancing hormones, and totally eliminating double chins.

◆ Take baths with Epsom salts. You'll love the relaxation time. Baths are a terrific way to lower high cortisol levels related to stress. The Epsom salts help soak away toxins near the skin. They provoke sweating as well. You can also use baking soda in your baths for detoxification. Baking soda helps neutralize acids and is a great remedy for itching skin.

◆ Bounce daily. An excellent physical exercise for detoxification is bouncing on a mini trampoline for at least five minutes every day, preferably in the morning. An alternative to the mini trampoline is a pair of KanGoo boots. The boots act like a trampoline or a pogo stick in that they give your body the same benefit as a mini trampoline, but you can actually jog around the neighborhood in them. Bouncing cleanses your lymph system by encouraging the lymph to get moving and release toxins from your body. As with any exercise, bouncing on either a mini trampoline or on the KanGoo boots also boosts cellular meta-bolism and tones your body. To learn more about KanGoo boots go to kangoojumps.com.

Skin-spiration

Susan's skin looked worn and tired. Her fibromyalgia was in remission, but the chronic autoimmune disorder had taken its toll on her skin. The pigmentation was uneven, and red blotches were everywhere. Then she started bouncing on her KanGoo boots every day. She loved how the bouncing lifted her endorphins, and thus her moods, and how it toned her legs. But the biggest surprise was how her skin changed. The pigmentation evened out, the redness disappeared, her blemishes abated, and she looked rested and youthful.

◆ Sweat. Sweating is one of your body's brilliant ways to release toxins. Sweat by taking hot baths, through aerobic exercise, and even through using saunas and steam rooms. But please go easy on the saunas and steam rooms. Stay in for short amounts of time—just enough time to get a sweat going. Too much intense heat can cause broken capillaries and exacerbate some skin conditions, such as rosacea. Be sure to shower after exercise and sauna or steam room visits to wash the toxins from your skin.

◆ Eat two or three servings of vegetables and fruits per meal. These powerhouses of nutrition help your body detoxify in two ways. First, they add purifying fiber to your diet. Second, they contain healthy antioxidants, which directly neutralize free radicals, which are a form of toxin in the body.

This program is a simple and easy way to incorporate detoxification into your day-to-day life. By detoxifying on an ongoing basis, you can avoid dramatic detoxification programs. Your daily detoxification program can be included as a part of your daily skin care regimen.

Other Detoxification Treatments

Many other techniques work to assist your body in detoxification. Some of these you can do daily or weekly. Use others less frequently. Here are some suggestions:

◆ Clay masks for your face. If your skin is oily, you can use a clay mask once or twice a week. Otherwise, use a clay mask to draw out toxins occasionally. Use clay masks after airplane travel, vacations, change of seasons, high-stress times, the holidays, and illness.

◆ Stretching. Yoga and other forms of stretching actually flush toxins out of muscles and body fat. Do two to three sessions of yoga or stretching per week to realize detoxifying benefits.

◆ Hot-towel wraps. Place a warm, wet towel over your face for 5 to 10 minutes to encourage gentle sweating. Be sure to leave a space for breathing. Wash your face afterwards to remove toxins.

◆ Chi machines. These remove toxins and waste products by gently wiggling the body from side to side. They can be rather pricey, so consider a chi machine as an investment that you'll use for years to come.

Body of Knowledge
Beware of detoxification programs that require fasting. Fasting causes the body to dump toxic compounds from body fat into the bloodstream. This impairs the liver's ability to detoxify them and results in the formation of toxic metabolites. The toxic metabolites are more harmful to your body than the original toxins. Plus, fasting always has a rebound effect of real—and not just water—weight gain.

◆ Body rolling. This exercise is an excellent way to remove toxins from the muscles. It relaxes your body just like a deep massage, but you can do body rolling at home. Body rolling is so relaxing that even your face will look more relaxed. To learn more, visit www.yamunabody-rolling.com or purchase the book *The Ultimate Body Rolling Workout* by Yamuna Zake, which is widely available (Broadway Books, 2003).

◆ Professional facials. This is an excellent way to detoxify the facial skin at the change of every season, or more frequently if you choose. Ask your skin care technician for a detoxification facial.

Start now with an ongoing plan to detoxify your body and you'll enjoy the benefits of having beautiful skin for the rest of your life.

The Least You Need to Know

◆ Everyone's body contains toxins that can detract from the skin's health and appearance.

◆ Many detoxification treatments are simple to perform, inexpensive, and take very little time.

◆ Follow the daily detoxification program to improve the condition of your skin.

◆ Use special detoxification treatments when needed for stress, illness, travel, vacations, and changing seasons.

Part **6**

Home Treatments for Your Skin

Infomercials regularly tout the latest skin care machine or system that is guaranteed to improve your skin in a wide variety of ways. Some of the hype is just that—hype. And some of the products can be quite helpful for at-home treatments. You'll learn which products are approved by the FDA and what they can and can't do.

Next we'll give you the information you need to get started with incorporating facial exercises into your regular routine. Facial exercises are here to stay, for good reason. They work. You'll find exercises to tone your forehead, the furrows between the eyebrows, and crow's feet around the eyes. You can also soothe the appearance of nasal labial folds and tighten sagging jowls and neck.

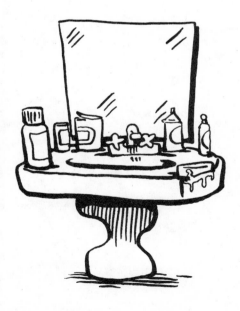

Chapter 24

Exercise: A Bonus for Your Skin

In This Chapter

- Exercising your body to benefit your skin
- Exercise program basics
- Enjoying recreational activities
- The Fountain of Youth exercises

If you're already exercising regularly—meaning three times a week for at least 30 minutes a session—you're already among the fitness elite. Your skin loves the exercise as much as your body and your mind do.

If you're among the 70 percent of adults living in the United States who don't exercise regularly, not only is your body deprived, so is your skin. The truth is this: It's much easier for you to have great skin if you are among the fitness elite.

Exercise takes planning and time. Quite simply, it's work. Physical work. But then, who ever said that having great skin is easy? However, if you're willing to put in the time and effort to exercise regularly, you'll love the results. In this chapter, you'll learn how and when to exercise in order to attain better skin.

Sweat Your Way to Great Skin

Your exercise habits show up in your skin. Sitting around and hugging the couch day after day is bad for your skin. Ditto for being too busy to exercise regularly. Without regular exercise, your skin becomes congested easily and is more likely to suffer from challenging skin conditions. The cell turnover rate is slower and your skin ages more quickly.

The benefits of regular exercise to your skin include the following:

- Increased cell turnover rate at any age
- Increased oxygenation of the skin
- Removal of cellular wastes through sweating
- Increased muscle tone in other parts of your body, which increases overall muscle tone—even in your face
- Skin less likely to be congested
- Imparts radiant glow to skin
- Improvement of overall skin tone and coloring
- Avoiding premature aging of skin
- Skin aging actually slows down

Exercise is a natural activity for human beings. If it weren't, you'd have been born with a sofa attached. Being sedentary is unnatural. Unfortunately, many people don't engage in regular exercise for a wide variety of reasons—they don't like it, they don't have the time, it's inconvenient, they're too tired, and because they just don't want to.

Historical Overview

Up until about 100 years ago, people were paid to exercise. Most jobs required manual labor. People moved all day long. Resting at home in the evening after work made sense.

Today, more people in the United States are paid to sit still than to do physical labor. In fact, today people need to pay to exercise. They sign up for membership at fitness facilities, they purchase exercise equipment, and they engage in recreation that requires gear, clothes, and equipment. It makes less sense to rest up after working all day than it does to get out and get moving in order to balance out sitting all day long.

Exercise is the single healthiest activity you can do for your body. It aids in the prevention of chronic diseases, such as diabetes, heart disease, high blood pressure, autoimmune diseases, obesity, and cancer. And certainly, what's good for your health is great for your face.

Body of Knowledge

The caveman and cavewoman walked six or seven miles a day just to find enough food to eat. Yet today we rarely require ourselves to walk six or seven miles for anything. But it wouldn't be a bad idea.

Getting Started

There's no time better than the present to embark on an exercise program. The best way to get started is to open up your daily agenda and schedule three one-hour sessions a week for the next four weeks. Choose a time that works for you—in the morning before work, during your lunch hour, or after work before dinner. You may find it easier to schedule weekend time, if that works for you and your family.

Next, plan which activities you are going to do. There are three types of exercise that a person needs to do on a regular basis.

- ◆ Aerobic or cardio. Do at least three 20-minute sessions every week. This is the time to work up a sweat. You'll strengthen your heart, increase physical endurance, and oxygenate your body. Choose from activities at the fitness center, such as aerobic classes, spinning, stationary bike, treadmill, elliptical machines, or swimming. You can also run, jog, or participate in sports such as racquetball or squash.

- ◆ Strength training. Schedule at least two 30-minute sessions per week, and it's preferable that you schedule two one-hour sessions. Strength training increases your muscle mass, reduces body fat percentage, gives your body shape and curves, and increases muscle tone. Choose from activities such as free weights, weight machines, Pilates, Magic Circle, stretch tubing, Fitball, and flex band workouts.

- ◆ Flexibility or stretching. Add at least 15 minutes three times a week for stretching. Stretching improves posture, reduces stress, helps prevent injury, and relaxes your muscles after exercise. You can practice yoga postures or regular stretching exercises. Stretching is especially wonderful after a long day's work. You'll feel refreshed and calm.

Those are the three basics and they need to be included in your exercise program. Your body will quickly adapt to your exercise routine, so when it feels as if your workout has become easy, it's time to raise the bar. Use heavier weights and increase the intensity of your aerobic or cardio exercise.

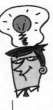

Skin-spiration

Using a pedometer can be a great way to get started with exercise awareness. A pedometer measures how many steps you take in a day. Ideally, you should take more than 10,000. When you first start wearing one, you may be surprised at how few steps you walk in a day. You may find yourself taking a walk around the block after dinner just to get in enough steps, which would be great.

Wrinkle Guard

Some sports don't count as exercise—at least not as the kind of exercise you need regularly. Golf, bowling, and boating don't do enough for you in terms of aerobics, muscle building, or flexibility. But they can be fun, so enjoy these sports in addition to the kinds of exercise that you and your skin require.

Recreation

Now for the fun part. We've just discussed a serious exercise program, all aspects of which are essential for the health of your body and the health of your skin. Now you can take it to the next level—to the level of recreation. Think of recreation as exercise with fun added in.

Take a friend or go by yourself. Choose an activity that brings joy to your heart. Go hiking, bicycling, snowshoeing, or cross-country skiing. Play tennis, basketball, racquetball, or volleyball. Go swimming or dancing. You can participate in walkathons, marathons, bikeathons, runs, and races.

Mood Enhancers

As you continue to exercise regularly, wonderful things happen. You'll have more energy and more stamina, and your moods will be lifted. Researchers explain that during aerobic exercise, the body releases endorphins, which give you the so-called runner's high. Only you don't need to be a runner to enjoy this wonderful feeling.

You'll find when you exercise that you enter a "zone." Some people describe this as a sense of "no time," others as a sense of "all time." When you enter the zone, you'll know. It feels delicious and you'll want to keep coming back for more. The zone is stress-free, relaxing, and joyous. It's also great for your skin and soothes any stressed facial muscles and expressions.

Fountain of Youth Exercises

Think of these exercises as a Fountain of Youth for your face. These five simple little exercises are great for your skin. They can make your face appear years younger, and they definitely rejuvenate your hormonal system. Within three months of doing these exercises, a person's double chin will vanish and the neck will seem elongated.

The Fountain of Youth exercises oxygenate the body and increase blood flow to the skin while increasing metabolic rate. They improve skin tone and help reduce the effects of aging. The exercises—especially the first one—are highly detoxifying and encourage the body to release toxins and waste products.

The Fountain of Youth exercises take less than 10 minutes a day. Many people like to do them first thing in the morning when they get out of bed. They give your body the feeling of having had a cup of coffee, but without needing to actually drink caffeine.

The exercises were first published in 1939 in a small book of 80 pages titled *Ancient Secrets of the Fountain of Youth* by Peter Kelder. Doubleday has since published a 301 page book with updated information, *Ancient Secrets of the Fountain of Youth, Part 2.*

If the exercises seem too strenuous at first, you can refer to the book *Ancient Secrets of the Fountain of Youth, Part 2* for starter exercises that assist in strengthening your body. In weeks, you'll easily be breezing through them.

Start by doing three repetitions of each Fountain of Youth exercise for the first week. Increase the number of repetitions for each exercise by two every week until you reach 21 repetitions, the full number recommended.

They can be performed any time of day, and many people do them twice a day, in the morning and late afternoon. It isn't necessary to do the exercises more than 21 times unless you are truly motivated to do so.

Exercise 1

Standing with arms out at your sides, turn toward your right hand. Start by making 3 complete revolutions with your arms and work up to 21. Go very slowly at first, being sure to stop if you feel a bit dizzy. Should you get dizzy, pick a spot on the wall and look at it until you feel clear-headed.

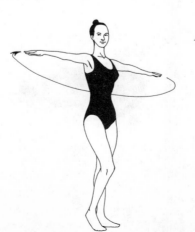

Fountain of Youth exercise 1.

Exercise 2

Lie flat on the floor, face up. Fully extend your arms along your sides, and place the palms of your hands against the floor, keeping the fingers close together. Then, raise your head off the floor, tucking your chin against your chest.

As you do this, lift your legs, knees straight, into a vertical position. If possible, let the legs extend back over the body, toward the head, but do not let your knees bend. Then slowly lower the head and the legs, knees straight, to the floor. Allow all the muscles to relax, continue breathing in the same rhythm. Breathe in deeply as you lift your legs and breathe out as you lower your legs. Start with 3 and work up to 21 repetitions.

Fountain of Youth exercise 2.

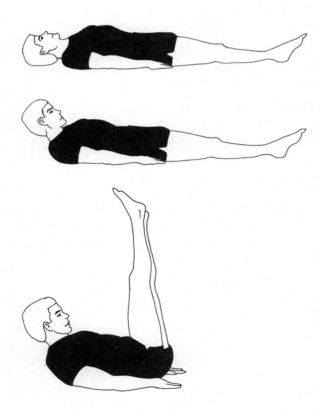

Exercise 3

Kneel on the floor with the body erect. Place your hands against the back of your thigh muscles or the small of your back, whichever is most comfortable. Incline your head and neck forward, tucking the chin against the chest. Then, move your head back as if to look at the back wall, arching the spine.

As you arch your neck backward, brace your arms and hands against the thighs or back for support. After arching, return to the original position and start the exercise all over again. Breathe in deeply as you arch the spine, breathe out as you return to an erect position. Start with 3, and work up to 21 repetitions.

Fountain of Youth exercise 3.

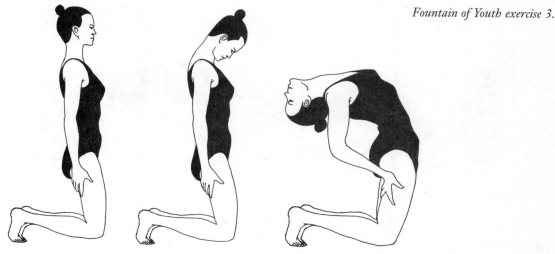

Exercise 4

Sit on the floor with your legs straight out in front of you and your feet about 12 inches apart. With the trunk of the body erect, place the palms of your hands on the floor alongside the buttocks. Then, tuck the chin forward against the chest. Now, drop the head backward as far as it will go. At the same time, raise your body so that the knees bend while the arms remain straight.

The trunk of your body will be in a straight line with the upper legs, horizontal to the floor. At this point, your body looks like a bench. Then, tense every muscle in the body, being sure to tighten the buttocks and stomach muscles. Finally, relax your muscles as you return to the original sitting position, and rest before repeating the procedure. Breathe in as you raise up, hold your breath as you tense the muscles, and breathe out completely as you come down. Start with 3, and work up to 21 repetitions.

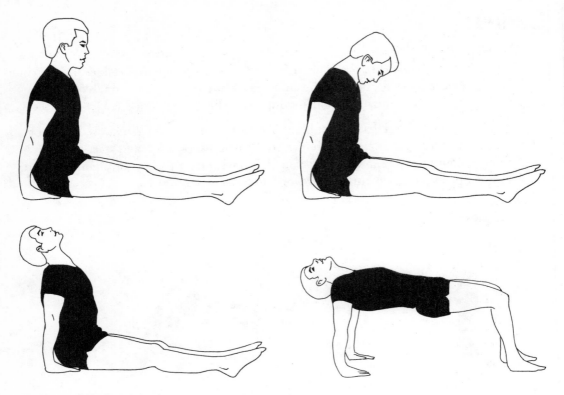

Fountain of Youth exercise 4.

Exercise 5

When you perform the fifth exercise, your body should be face down facing toward the floor. Support your body with your hands, palms down against the floor, and the toes in a flexed position. Throughout this exercise, the hands and feet don't move. Start with your arms perpendicular to the floor, with the spine arched and head back, such that the body near the hips seems to sag toward the floor.

Now, start moving your head toward your chest. Then, bending at the waist, bring the body up into an inverted *V.* Your hips are now higher than the rest of your body. At the same time, bring the chin forward, tucking it against the chest. Breathe in deeply as you raise the body, breathe out fully as you lower it. Start with 3 repetitions and increase to 21.

The secret to these exercises is to do them faithfully every day. Sure, you could miss one day a week, but as you begin to see results, you won't ever want to stop. Your friends may ask if you've lost weight as they notice your slimmer chin, neck, and jaw line. This is the only exercise we know of that eliminates a double chin, and the only one that also effectively balances hormones and reverses the effects of aging.

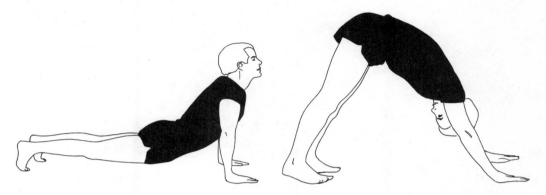

Fountain of Youth exercise 5.

The Least You Need to Know

◆ Regular exercise is a great tonic and treatment for your skin.

◆ Include aerobic, strength, and flexibility training in your weekly exercise program.

◆ Find athletic recreation that you enjoy and do it often.

◆ Schedule your exercise sessions into your daily agenda to assure that you make time to exercise every week.

◆ Do the Fountain of Youth exercises every day to balance hormones, eliminate a double chin, and keep your skin vibrant.

25

Home and Salon Skin-Treatment Machines

In This Chapter

- ◆ Using skin-treatment machines
- ◆ Weighing the pros and cons of each device
- ◆ Doing no harm
- ◆ Expecting realistic results

Perhaps you've seen the infomercials espousing home-use skin care machines and gadgets that claim to dramatically improve the appearance of your skin. The before and after pictures are impressive, and they have to be. After all, the purpose of the sales pitch is to motivate you to rush to the phone and place an order immediately.

Skin care technicians often use similar skin treatment machines for facials and other services. But are the machines hype or help? Are they merely feel-good devices that provide little more than cosmetic value, or do they actually make a significant difference in the condition of your skin?

In this chapter, you'll learn the facts about the pros and cons of oxygen facials, facial exercisers, microdermabrasion, ultrasound machines, light therapy, and skin-tag removers.

FDA Approval

As we write this chapter, the Food and Drug Administration is carefully scrutinizing many of the machines and devices mentioned here. The devices in question, such as facial exercisers, are designed to affect the structure or function of the body. Because of that, the machines need to have FDA approval before they can be offered for sale.

But whether or not the FDA has sanctioned the machines, they're flooding the market, the Internet, and late-night infomercials. Before you purchase one of these devices, be aware that the FDA is on the lookout for companies selling unapproved devices and may shut them down, in which case you'd be left without customer service and warranty replacements.

The only way for you to be protected as a consumer is to ask salespeople if the device has received FDA approval. Do your best to be fully informed before making your purchasing decision.

We feel that skin care treatment devices are here to stay. We also know that people will use the devices whether or not the FDA approves them. We'll give you the information about them in this chapter, and let you be the judge.

Oxygen Facials

Your skin receives benefits from oxygen every time you breathe. And since the air around you is composed of 18 percent oxygen, you receive adequate oxygen to sustain life and remain healthy. Your skin benefits with your every breath.

It's unlikely that you need more oxygen at the surface of your skin or that the oxygen can significantly improve it. However, oxygen facials, which deliver regular oxygen as a gas mist or in the form of a facial cream, have become exceedingly popular. The effectiveness of oxygen facials has never been scientifically tested.

According to product claims, oxygen facials …

- ◆ Improve the appearance of the skin.
- ◆ Eliminate redness and irritation.
- ◆ Fight bacteria associated with acne.

- Soothe the appearance of skin irritated by microdermabrasion, laser, and acid peels.

- Boost collagen and elastin synthesis and formation.

- Include hydrogen peroxide cream, which helps put water and oxygen into the skin.

The Pros:

Any facial is soothing, feels good, and tends to calm irritated skin.

The Cons:

None of these claims are substantiated by research.

Oxygen applied to the skin as a mist or in combination with hydrogen peroxide cream can increase the amount of free radicals on the skin and actually do damage that ages the skin. Hydrogen peroxide is a free radical, so beware.

Dermatologists and health experts warn that the oxygen is more likely to hurt your skin than help it.

Oxygen facials seem to be more hype than help. A regular facial can produce results similar to the claims without any undue or unnecessary risk. The cost in most cities for an oxygen facial is $60 not including tip. However, expect to pay more at resorts, spas, hotels, and big cities.

CAUTION

Wrinkle Guard

Oxygen facials aren't for everyone. If you have sensitive skin, your skin could become red and inflamed after the procedure. If this happens, immediately before you leave the studio, ask for a soothing and healing treatment to reverse the damage and inflammation. Don't leave the studio with a face that's burning or red.

Facial Flex Bands

These very simple devices are registered as a medical product and are clinically proven effective as a facial exerciser. The band is placed in the corners of the mouth. You work your mouth and cheek muscles to compress and release against the force of an elastic resistance band, doing 100 to 120 repetitions each morning and evening.

According to product claims, facial flex bands …

- Recapture the facial contours of youth.

- Strengthen and tone the muscles of the face, neck, and chin.

◆ Are shown by independent studies to provide a 32 percent increase in facial firmness and a 250 percent increase in facial muscle strength after eight weeks of use.

The Pros:

Research indicates this device is effective.

The Cons:

The device requires continued use to maintain results.

Before you decide to purchase a facial flex band, ask to see before and after photos and personal testimonials. If you're satisfied with what you see and decide to purchase, ask for a money-back guarantee. Purchase price is about $65.

Wrinkle Guard

Experts don't agree about the value of facial exercisers or facial exercises. The facial muscles aren't long muscles, such as the legs, arms, and abdomen, and some think they don't respond to exercise. But many people who do facial exercises swear by them. They may work very well for you or not. To find out, you'll need to try them for yourself.

Facial Exercisers

These devices give you a nonsurgical face-lift by using light electrical currents to passively contract the muscles of the face and neck. The contractions cause the muscles to tighten, as if through exercise. Facial exercisers are widely available for home use through the Internet and infomercials.

Skin-spiration

The renowned dermatologist and author Dr. Nicholas Perricone, author of *The Wrinkle Cure*, is enthusiastic about facial exercisers. Dr. Perricone's version of the facial exerciser is now being evaluated by the FDA and will be available when approved.

Salons offer facial exercise treatments using more sophisticated and expensive equipment. Single sessions at the salon can range from $50 to over $100. Home equipment prices start at about $100 and go up to about $200.

Many dermatologists recommend the use of home facial exercisers. They agree that the facial muscles get shorter and rounder after use, which is a characteristic of a younger face.

Many dermatologists disagree. There are no studies to support the claims that facial exercisers work. Certainly, electrical currents can stimulate the muscles, as electrical stimulation is used to help bones heal and promote skin growth. But many experts state that facial exercisers cannot deliver a nonsurgical face-lift.

According to product claims, facial exercisers …

- Provide a nonsurgical face-lift with regular use.

- Are safe to use.

- Reduce double chins, forehead furrows, crow's feet, sagging jaw line, and creases under the eyes.

- Don't hurt.

Wrinkle Guard

Protect your wallet as you work to improve your skin. Be sure your purchase comes with a full money-back guarantee with no questions asked. Don't be embarrassed to return a product that doesn't perform as you expected.

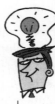

Skin-spiration

Many Hollywood stars are reported to visit skin care specialists for facial exerciser sessions prior to walks on the red carpet at award ceremonies.

The Pros:

Facial exercisers are inexpensive compared to a surgical face-lift.

Some dermatologists and skin care technicians advocate their use.

They can be highly effective for tightening muscles and reducing lines, wrinkle, and sags.

The Cons:

Few facial exercisers are approved by the FDA.

The devices can hurt and sting the face.

They can create broken capillaries on the surface of skin.

The device needs to be used two to three times a week to maintain results. Sessions take about 15 minutes.

They aren't effective for exceedingly loose or sagging skin.

Before you purchase a facial exerciser, talk with someone who has actually used one and not only the person selling the device. Find out if the person is happy with the results and also ask if he or she experienced any bad reactions or negative results.

Microdermabrasion for Personal and Salon Use

Think of microdermabrasion as polish taken to the extreme. It's a deep skin scrub performed using finely ground mineral crystals. You can have microdermabrasion done at a salon and intense microdermabrasion performed at a doctor's office. You can also purchase a home-use microdermabrasion machine and perform this treatment for yourself. The machine is far more gentle than those used by professionals.

Even some skin care lines are now offering exfoliating scrubs that contain the mineral crystals. The products are called microdermabrasion scrubs, but they're really exfoliating scrubs and simply can't produce the same results as microdermabrasion. But they work well as exfoliants.

The treatment temporarily improves the appearance of your skin. It has little to no effect in removing deeply colored pigmentation, but it minimizes the appearance of fine lines and increases skin cell turnover rate. The salon procedure takes about 20 to 30 minutes and leaves skin with a healthy glow, so it can be done on a person's lunch hour. Most salons recommend a series of 5 to 10 treatments at two- to three-week intervals. Usually, results are seen after four or five sessions.

The term "lunchtime peel" initially referred to a light glycolic peel done by an aesthetician. The idea is that a person could have a peel done during the lunch hour and return directly to work without any redness or inflammation.

Wrinkle Guard

Some experts say that inflammation from such procedures as microdermabrasion, peels, and lasers, plus topical treatments such as Retin-A and Renova causes the skin to regenerate itself and that these treatments improve skin tone and texture. Be sure never to overdo such procedures, but a little intentional inflammation can be good for your skin. Other leading experts recommend lowering bodily inflammation levels through a proper diet and by making lifestyle changes. Doing this can help your skin avoid sagging and wrinkles. So a little intentional inflammation is great, but reduce inflammation as much as possible in other ways.

Microdermabrasion can cause redness and irritation, especially if done in conjunction with a light glycolic peel. In addition, mistakes can occur. A skin care technician can get too aggressive, and so can a person using a home machine. You could end up with open lesions and possibly, scarring. Don't use microdermabrasion if you are prone to cold sores—herpes simplex—as microdermabrasion can trigger an outbreak, and never use it on open sores or blemishes.

If you purchase a home microdermabrasion device, be very gentle and go slow. Learn how your skin reacts to microdermabrasion. If you have sensitive skin, or any kind of skin condition, be sure you don't make it worse.

According to product claims, microdermabrasion …

- Reduces sun damage.
- Brightens complexions.
- Is safe.
- Eliminates early signs of aging.
- Improves dull, oily, or leathery skin textures.
- Contracts large pores.
- Reduces fine lines.
- Smoothes mild pigmentation irregularities.
- Requires no downtime or recovery time.

The Pros:

After four to five sessions, the skin will appear fresher and more radiant.

The procedure can be done at home or at the salon.

It's safe when used properly and gently.

The Cons:

Aggressive use can lead to scarring and open lesions.

The procedure can trigger a herpes simplex outbreak.

It's temporary and requires maintenance to sustain results.

Microdermabrasion can be beneficial when used correctly. Stop using it if your skin gets red, flaky, or dry. For home use, follow the directions carefully and keep in mind that with this type of procedure, less is often more.

Ultrasound Machines

One of the most recently developed facial care devices is an ultrasound machine. This skin care system uses low-frequency sound waves to improve the appearance of skin.

The devices use a liquid medium, such as water or gel, to exfoliate the skin and give deeper penetration to skin care products.

The exfoliation is accomplished through a process called cavitation, in which the water or gel molecules are driven by the low-frequency sound waves to spin rapidly. Cavitation removes dead skin cells safely and gently with no inflammation. This type of exfoliation is a scrub, albeit a sophisticated scrub. The same cautions apply as for all scrub exfoliants. Go slow, go easy, and don't expect miracles.

Ultrasound skin care machines are available for home use. Salons also offer ultrasound facials, using similar equipment.

According to product claims, ultrasound machines …

- Reduce fine lines, wrinkles, age spots, and scars.
- Exfoliate skin, removing dead skin cells.
- Stimulate new skin cell growth.
- Give skin a youthful texture and appearance.
- Make skin care products penetrate into deep skin layers.
- Repair sun-damaged skin.
- Stimulate new collagen production.

The Pros:

Devices are safe when used properly per directions.

Use of machines improves the skin's appearance.

The Cons:

They need to be used regularly to maintain results.

Ultrasound use can be overdone.

You need to avoid using the devices if you have any skin disease, such as herpes simplex, skin cancer, or melanoma.

They're not advised for sensitive skin.

Don't use the devices if you have a pacemaker, or implanted wires or appliances.

It's doubtful that ultrasound can help skin care products penetrate more deeply into the skin. The product manufacturers don't cite research studies that prove this.

The product claims are unrealistic, given the limited capabilities of any noninvasive skin care treatments. However, your skin may get clearer and more radiant skin with continued use.

Light Therapy

Using light is helpful for some people in correcting the skin conditions of psoriasis and acne. You can purchase light therapy equipment for home use, or visit a salon or dermatologist for light treatments.

The lights used in light therapy for psoriasis simulate natural sunlight, so it counts as sun exposure. Be sure to wear sunscreen. Use the light boxes for 15-minute sessions two to three times a week for a duration of 30 treatments. Experts theorize that the ultraviolet rays decrease the cells' overactive production rates.

Skin-spiration

New light therapy treatments are discovered frequently. If you have a skin condition, ask your dermatologist if light therapy could be beneficial.

Light therapy for acne doesn't require UV radiation, but instead uses light of red and blue wavelengths. Both wavelengths are thought to attack p. acne bacteria, and thus promote healing. Sit under the lights for 15-minute sessions every day for 12 weeks to determine if light therapy will clear up your acne.

According to product claims, light therapy …

 ♦ Can be helpful in reducing the symptoms of psoriasis and acne.

The Pros:

 The procedure has been shown to be effective for some people.

The Cons:

 It may not work for everyone.

 You must use sunscreen for psoriasis treatments.

 Fair-haired people—those more susceptible to skin cancer—may need to limit exposure to UV light, even with the use of sunscreen.

Ask your dermatologist or doctor if light therapy can work for your skin condition. If so, a light box could be a very good investment.

VascuLyse Machines

These machines use radio frequencies to eliminate annoying spots and tags on the skin. They work on spider veins, ruby red veins, blotchiness, *couperose* skin, *telangiectasia*, and skin tags.

The machines use a mild current to induce coagulation within the distended capillary. Sessions range between 5 and 15 minutes in length and are mostly done in a salon. Most skin concerns can be corrected within one to three sessions.

The treatment can be slightly painful and results are usually noticeable within seven days. The clotted blood under the skin after a treatment is absorbed into the body within a couple days and removed through the body's internal elimination system.

Clarifying Words

Couperose describes skin that has dilated or broken capillaries. **Telangiectasia** is the chronic dilation of groups of capillaries that cause elevated dark red blotches on the skin.

According to product claims, VascuLyse machines ...

- Eliminate skin tags, spider veins, couperose skin, blotchiness, ruby red veins, and telangiectasia.

- Require only one to three sessions.

- Don't require repeat treatments once the imperfection is removed.

The Pros:

The device is noninvasive.

It's effective when used properly.

The Cons:

You should expect some post-treatment scabbing from skin tags and bruising.

The procedure may not correct all situations.

You can't do these procedures on yourself.

VascuLyse machines are effective for what they claim to do, but the FDA has not approved all of the machines. Ask your skin care technician about his or her experience using the machine with clients before you schedule an appointment.

The Least You Need to Know

- Skin care machines and other devices are popular for improving the appearance of the skin.

- Use caution when using any electrical device on your face to avoid harmful mistakes.

- Be gentle when using exfoliating machines to avoid irritation and inflammation, which actually damage the skin.

- Check out all product claims to verify accuracy and ask for a money-back guarantee before you purchase.

Chapter 26

Facial Exercises

In This Chapter

- Using facial exercises to improve appearance
- Eliminating bad habits that cause wrinkles
- Exercises that target problem areas
- Tips for relaxing the face

Good muscle tone is highly prized and desired. Both men and women want muscle definition in their thighs, abdominals, and upper arms. Strong muscles indicate vigor, energy, and long hours at the fitness center. Good muscle tone doesn't just happen naturally. It takes work.

But what about exercising one's face? For men and women alike, good facial muscle tone implies no sagging or loose skin and few wrinkles. Well-exercised facial muscles are shorter, tighter, and rounder, giving the face a more youthful, relaxed appearance. Having toned facial muscles might even stave off the desire for facial surgery. Just like body toning, having toned facial muscles takes work—and continued maintenance.

In this chapter, you'll learn the truth about the benefits and limitations of facial exercises. Included are several easy-to-do exercises to tone the most common wrinkle areas of your face.

The Jury's Still Out

Facial exercises seem to pull experts into two camps. One side says, "Rubbish. The exercises can't do anything except create more wrinkles. They're a total waste of time." On the other side are avowed believers whose faces belie their age. They look great without resorting to plastic surgery.

Because there is absolutely no consensus among the experts, the only way to tell if facial exercises will work for you is to give them a try.

Facial exercises may help you look younger, but they aren't a cure-all. They can't reverse sun damage and they aren't considered to be a substitute for plastic surgery. If a person has skin with lots of sagging, the exercises can't lift or shrink the loose skin adequately. Plastic surgery is still necessary to reduce sags and loose skin in order to look younger.

However, the exercises *do* have some benefits. Facial exercises can lift eyebrows, reduce furrows between the eyebrows, and lighten crow's feet. For some people, they can even eliminate double chins and jowls. Overall, you can look younger.

But there's a catch. And it's a big catch. There's a price to pay, and that price is actually doing the exercises. At first, you'll need to do them three to five times a week for three months to see results. At the end of three months, if you compare a before and after photo, you'll readily see the difference.

Skin-spiration

If you get started on a program of facial exercises and then stop doing them, don't despair. Restart your program and you'll find that your facial muscles respond more quickly to the exercises than before. This is true for all the muscles in your body, not just your face.

The rest of the catch is this: You'll need to continue doing the facial exercises once or twice a week to maintain your results. For some people, it's tough to maintain that kind of commitment. For others, it's worth it.

Many of the facial exercises can be performed while you are doing something else, such as driving in the car, or talking on the phone. But some require more concentration. For those, you need to sit down and focus on actually feeling the muscles contract and fatigue, just as you would if you were building muscles at a fitness center.

Before You Begin

Now is the time to break repetitive motion bad habits that may be causing facial wrinkles and sagging. If you keep doing the very things that created the wrinkles in the first place, the exercises will have little to no value. The following habits could be causing your existing wrinkles:

- Whistling. If you whistle while you work, it shows in wrinkles around your lips and mouth.

- Smoking. The telltale signs of smoking are smoker's lips—fine vertical lines surrounding the lips.

- Squinting. If you need glasses, then wear glasses. Squinting accelerates the formation of crow's feet. If you squint when you go out in the sunshine, make it a habit to wear sunglasses when outdoors.

- Scowling. This action causes the space between your eyebrows to furrow. As they become etched into your facial expression, you can look permanently angry or upset.

- Frowning. Frowning too often makes the corners of your mouth turn down. One solution? Smile frequently.

- Smiling. This can also give you facial lines, but they tend to be far more acceptable than frown lines. Don't sweat the smile lines, they make you look happy, and that's always welcome.

One advantage of doing facial exercises is that you'll become more aware of your unconscious facial expressions like the ones mentioned previously. You'll be able to correct them instinctively. The result—you'll look more rested and relaxed.

Wrinkle Guard

Facial exercise systems claim the exercises won't give you more wrinkles if you do them correctly. But this statement is controversial among some skin care experts. Be sure you aren't squinting your eyes or forming wrinkles as you do the exercises. That's a sure way to tell if you are doing the exercise incorrectly. Use a mirror to make sure you aren't etching new wrinkles in a effort to eliminate others.

Getting Started

The best way to get started is first of all to decide that yes, you are committed to learning about facial exercises and to doing them faithfully for at least three months. Check out the exercises that follow as starter exercises. Yes, they'll make a big difference. But they aren't a comprehensive system of facial exercises. We've chosen to give you exercises to correct the most common wrinkles and sags.

Wrinkle Guard

Don't attempt facial exercises if you have a limited range of movement in your neck, if you are under chiropractic care, or if you are undergoing intensive dental work.

Next, go to the bookstore or go online and select a facial exercise system to work with. If you can find a video or CD of the exercises, that can be helpful for learning the correct way to do them. A favorite book is Carole Maggio's *Facercise* (Perigree, 2002).

Next, look at your daily agenda and schedule three to five sessions every week for three months. The facial exercises don't take a lot of time, so you'll only need to set aside 20 to 30 minutes for each session.

Lastly, have realistic expectations. Remember that change from exercise is gradual and it takes time to tighten up muscles and get them firm again. You already know how difficult it can be to regain a flat stomach after years of inactivity. Give yourself the luxury of time and be patient. View the whole process with a loving attitude.

The Exercises

As you perform facial exercises, you'll learn how to control the muscles of the face. This is a very positive aspect of facial exercises. You learn how to move your facial muscles correctly to create a relaxed and unlined face. The more you do the exercises, the more unconscious this becomes, and soon your face will naturally look relaxed because you have programmed your facial muscles to move correctly.

Think of this as similar to body movement training, such as core training, Pilates, yoga, or ballet. After time, your body naturally stays more erect, your posture improves, and you hold your stomach in as you move. The same thing happens with your skin after you start doing facial exercises regularly. You'll learn how to smile, how to avoid scowling, and how to avoid wrinkling your forehead.

As you perform each exercise, be sure that you don't grimace or squint. Use a mirror so that you can make sure you are doing the exercises correctly. Doing them in a haphazard way is a waste of time and can give you unwanted results.

Smoothing Your Neck

One of the first things to make a person look older, even in your 20s and 30s, is the beginnings of a double chin. You can change this quickly.

The best exercises for eliminating a double chin are the Fountain of Youth exercises in Chapter 24. Do these exercises every day and within three months, any trace of a double chin will vanish. Keep doing the exercises to maintain a smooth and taut neck.

Another exercise that relaxes the neck muscles and soothes tension are neck rolls. While sitting or standing, move your chin toward your chest and then roll your neck toward your right shoulder, then toward your back, then over your left shoulder and back around to the front. Do this very slowly three times in each direction. As you do this exercise, you'll feel the muscles of your neck and shoulders relax. This exercise eases stress on your face.

Mouth and Chin

Here are two powerful exercises that tighten and tone the entire mouth, tongue, and chin area.

The first comes from yoga and is called "Lion." Sit comfortably, with your hands on your knees. Exhale until your lungs are emptied of air. Then open up your eyes and mouth widely. Stick out your tongue as far as possible and hold for 6 to 10 seconds. Relax, and repeat four more times.

Look in a mirror to be sure that the nasal labial fold between your nose and mouth is totally smooth. When you open your eyes widely, your forehead shouldn't wrinkle. Be sure to hold your breath as you do the exercise, as this also helps tone the muscles.

This exercise tones your neck and chin, and helps soften the nasal labial folds and the entire mouth area. You are also strengthening and stretching the muscles surrounding the *vagus nerve*, which is an important part of good digestion and overall health.

The second exercise is called "The Xs." When sitting or standing, pronounce the letter X in a very exaggerated way. You'll notice that your chin juts forward. Hold this for four to six seconds, then release. Repeat four more times, for a total of five repetitions. "The Xs" tones the neck and chin, relaxes the jaw, and helps shrink jowls.

Clarifying Words

The **vagus nerve** is also known as the wandering nerve. It originates in the brain and runs along the front of the neck, then down into the esophagus, heart, and stomach. Important for swallowing, digestion, hearing, and heart function, dysfunction of the vagus nerve can result in ringing in the ears, heart palpitations, heartburn, and acid reflux.

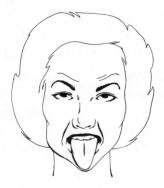

The Lion exercise.

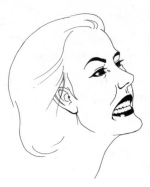

The Xs exercise.

Eyebrow Lifter

You can easily lift your eyebrows by exercising the forehead muscles. The exercise shortens and tightens the forehead muscles. This creates more space between your eyes and your eyebrows. Women will have more room to apply eye shadow, while men will simply look years younger.

Place your fingers along and just below the eyebrows. Gently press your fingers up toward your hairline. At the same time, scowl and try to push the fingers down. This is a resistance-type exercise. Hold for four to six seconds, then release. Do five repetitions.

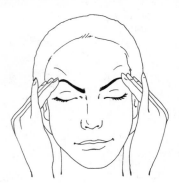

Eyebrow and forehead lifter.

As you do this exercise, look in the mirror to make sure you aren't creating wrinkles on your forehead or furrows between your borrows. The skin should be smooth. As you do this exercise over time, your forehead muscles will become stronger. Even if your eyebrows move up 1/16th of an inch, you'll see a big improvement in the youthfulness of your face.

Furrows Between Eyebrows

Certainly these furrows are the most frustrating lines to get rid of—and they come from being frustrated. Or angry. Or impatient.

First and foremost, you need to stop scowling. Yes, it's easier said than done. But as you do this exercise, you'll develop more awareness of the muscles in your face and you'll be able to control your facial expression.

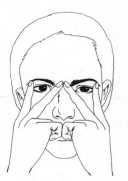

Exercise for furrows between brows.

Place the tips of your index fingers along both sides of the bridge of your nose, so that the tips are touching each other. Contract your forehead muscles upward against the resistance of your fingers. Hold for four to six seconds. Then relax. Do five repetitions in all.

Lips and Mouth

This exercise helps keep your lips full and plump and helps erase lines around the mouth. It also soothes nasal labial folds. It's called "Doing *O*s." Be sure to look in a mirror as you do this exercise to make sure you aren't creating wrinkling.

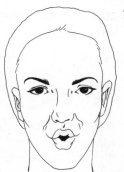

The Os exercise.

Say *"O"* in an exaggerated way, while you try to smile. Hold for four to six seconds, then relax. Do five repetitions.

Crow's Feet

This exercise helps eliminate crow's feet and repatterns your facial movements to avoid the squinting that causes crow's feet.

Crow's feet exercise.

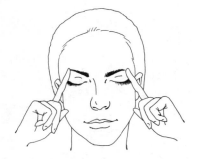

Place your index fingers at the outside of the eye. The top third of the index finger rests between the end of the eyebrow and the edge of the eye. Press gently. Then close your eyes. You'll feel a slight pull inward. Resist letting your fingers move. Hold for four to six seconds. Do five repetitions.

The exercises in this chapter are but a small sampling of the many exercises available. If you see results from these exercises, you may want to explore other approaches and exercise systems.

Relaxing the Face

Sometimes, you may want to look more relaxed and pampered. Wouldn't it be great to simply iron away the stress that shows up in your face? Here are several ways to essentially achieve the same results:

◆ Continue to do the facial exercises described in this chapter. Your face will become repatterned and you'll naturally look more relaxed.

◆ Massage. This can be facial massage or body massage.

◆ Professional facials. You'll leave the spa or salon looking as if you just returned home from vacation.

- Acupressure, acupuncture, and shiatsu treatments. These treatments are excellent for overall relaxation and can also be used specifically for the face. You'll definitely look refreshed and your face will be relaxed. A terrific temporary wrinkle reducer.

- Yoga classes or yoga sessions. Yoga is soothing for the body and also for the face. You'll look more relaxed and your expression lines will be soothed, at least temporarily.

If you don't have time for these, simply lying in bed with your feet up for 15 to 20 minutes can help freshen and relax your face.

The Least You Need to Know

- Properly done, facial exercises can restore a youthful appearance to your face.

- Facial exercises can't totally eliminate the effects of lifelong bad habits and repetitive movements.

- Facial exercises won't be totally effective for heavily sagging skin, sun damage, and smoker's lips.

- Use the facial exercises in this chapter to perk up your appearance and minimize problem areas.

Part  Professional Treatments

Facials feel wonderful. They're relaxing and they make you feel good. Better yet, they make your skin look great. The same is true of the many skin care treatments available through salons and spas. You'll discover what kinds of facials and treatments are best for your specific genetic skin type.

Medical doctors and paramedical professionals offer skin procedures designed to improve the appearance of your skin. We can't tell you they are always relaxing and soothing, but they'll make your skin look relaxed and soothed. Sometimes you'll get results right away, and sometimes you need to wait until you heal. And finally, you'll learn what to expect from plastic surgery, how to choose a surgeon, and how to plan for recovery.

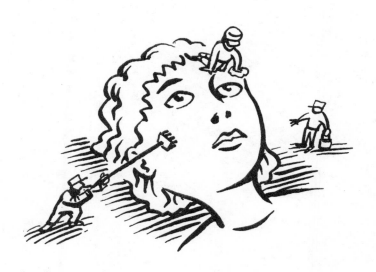

27

All About Skin Care Professionals

In This Chapter

- ◆ The roles of skin care professionals
- ◆ Learning what different professionals offer
- ◆ Licensing and state regulations
- ◆ Choosing the right professional for your skin care needs

A vast world of skin care professionals is available to assist you with your skin and its appearance. These professionals know how important your skin is to you, and their mission is to help you reach your goal of better skin.

Professionals can be found at the department store skin care counters, at salons and spas, at the dermatologist's office, and at the plastic surgeon's office. Your job is to find the best professional to meet your needs, and we're here to help you do that.

In this chapter, you'll learn all about the skin care profession. We'll clue you in on how each type of professional can help you. You'll understand the nuances of their educational requirements, their licensing restrictions, and the extent of their services.

The Perfect Person for the Job

If you leaf through the yellow pages, you can find hundreds of skin care specialists depending on the size of the city you live in. Notice how many entries you find listed under beauty salons, day spas, dermatologists, and plastic surgeons. Skin care is big business—even in a small city.

Choosing the right skin care professional begins with knowing what each can and can't do for you and your skin. In the sections that follow, you'll find information on each type. Licensing requirements and regulations vary from state to state, so the information may be slightly different where you live.

For example, some states, such as Colorado, are attempting to eliminate licensing for certain skin care technicians. Other states, such as Utah, just recently began to license skin and nail technicians. As best you can, engage the services of a professional who is licensed by your state. That means they have completed an educational program for becoming an aesthetician of about 600 hours, received a diploma, and passed a state licensing examination. You should be able to find out the details of your state's requirements for licensing with a little bit of research.

State licensing doesn't require that skin care technicians have a medical background or one in health or wellness. But these can be useful in treating skin. If this is important to you, work with skin care technicians who are also nurses or who have degrees in wellness or health.

You need to use caution when choosing a skin care specialist. Some are excellent, others are good, and some aren't highly skilled or capable. To find an esthetician, ask your friends and colleagues for referrals. If you plan to use skin care services at a spa, studio, or clinic, request that you are scheduled with their best esthetician. You simply don't want any mistakes.

Wrinkle Guard

Not all skin care specialists carefully follow the guidelines for their licensing. If someone offers to perform a service that seems beyond the scope of his or her practice, pass on it. An example would be an eye surgeon or ophthalmologist who suggests performing laser surgery to remove dark pigmentation on your face. His or her medical training isn't for skin care, but rather for eye care. Instead, go to a professional who specializes in laser dermatology.

Makeup Artists

Anyone can put out a shingle and print up a business card that reads, "Makeup Artist." In general, makeup artists aren't regulated or licensed in any state. If a makeup artist works for theatrical companies, the media, or the movies, he or she needs to join a union.

Most states require that anyone who touches another person's face, hair, or body needs to be licensed. Makeup artists bypass this requirement by using tools, such as brushes and sponges, to apply makeup; therefore, their fingers don't touch the client's face.

Makeup artists are often called upon to do the makeup of brides and the entire wedding party. They also work closely with professional photographers for personal portraits or modeling shots.

You may want to engage the services of a makeup artist before a special party or event. Also consider updating your look every couple of years. If you are entering the workforce, changing careers, or moving in or out of a long-term relationship, a new and updated look may give you an increased sense of confidence and strength.

If you are undergoing a life-changing event, such as losing weight, an updated makeup look can help you view yourself as if you had already reached your ideal size. The same applies if you've completed a dramatic change. For example, if you've just had plastic surgery, updated makeup will compliment the updated contours of your face.

Plus, it's plain old "girlish" fun to have your makeup done. Be sure you learn new techniques and color placement as the artist does your face so you can duplicate the look when you return home.

You can find makeup artists in the phone book, usually under the heading "Makeup Artists." Many skin care lines offer free makeovers at the department stores. You can schedule time with a makeup artist; sometimes you are expected to purchase a product and sometimes not. Check before you sign up.

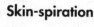 **Skin-spiration**

Skin care salons and spas often offer makeup sessions and are sometimes able to accommodate whole wedding parties the morning of the big event.

Estheticians

Also known as cosmeticians and skin care technicians, estheticians are professionals who have attended beauty school and focused their training in skin care. They have diplomas signifying they have taken 600 to 800 hours of classes (actual hours equaling about a six month course) in skin care, and they've passed a state board exam.

An esthetician is qualified to give you a facial, apply makeup, and perform hair removal in the forms of waxing and tweezing. They can also apply glycolic acid peels and microdermabrasion. Some states, such as Utah and Colorado now require extra training hours for an esthetician to become certified as a practitioner of glycolic acid peels and microdermabrasion.

Esthetician should know all about the skin and have good experience in working with all skin types. They often have the inside scoop on which products work best, and know numerous tricks of the trade. They can advise you on what skin products to use to get the best results, and they can design a home-care program that meets your lifestyle needs.

Skin-spiration

Your skin cells turn over every 30 days or so. To get the best results from facials, monthly visits are your very best choice. If that's too frequent for you or your budget, plan on having a facial quarterly as the seasons change. And when you find an esthetician who understands you and your skin, rejoice and continue to use her services.

They may also sell skin care products, but if their price point is too high for you, ask what drugstore products they would recommend. A good esthetician is more interested in your having a good at-home program, regardless of where you purchase the products.

Find estheticians at skin care salons, hair salons, skin studios, and occasionally at department stores. Expect to pay $60 and up for a facial.

Cosmetologists

Cosmetologists have spent many hours in class learning about hair. They can cut, style, bleach, dye, and perm. They can do nails. They can also do facials, although they have less training in skin care.

A cosmetologist can perform all the functions of an esthetician. Today, most professionals choose an area of specialization, such as hair, nails, or skin. But at small salons and in small towns, one person may do all three.

If you find a cosmetologist who is great with facials and skin care, wonderful. Keep using his or her services.

Permanent Makeup

Perhaps you've considered getting some tattoos—as in permanent makeup. Permanent eyeliner, eyebrows, and even lipstick are becoming more and more popular, especially with fair-haired people, and with both men and women.

Interestingly enough, even though tattoo artists poke through the skin, they aren't regulated by the states. Anyone can buy a machine and start doing permanent makeup. So be careful when choosing an artist, and find someone you can trust.

Here's what to look for:

◆ Length of time doing permanent makeup

◆ Experience

◆ Photos of their work

◆ Cleanliness of the studio

◆ Use of new—not just sterilized—needles for each session

Ask the makeup artist to use a light touch. Remember, you'll live with permanent makeup for the rest of your life. Anything too dark today could look garish and embarrassing in your 50s and 60s.

Paramedical Estheticians

An esthetician with more training hours can become qualified to work within a medical practice. They're known as paramedical estheticians. You'll find them working at medical skin care centers and dermatologist's offices.

But, as of now, there isn't a beauty school that trains paramedical estheticians. Nor are there any state certifications. A few schools offer advanced training for estheticians. Right now, the name medical esthetician can mean anything, so look beyond the title to the person's experience and background.

Paramedical estheticians can be qualified to work with lasers or freeze a keratosis (build up of dry skin). They can give you a chemical peel with glycolic acid. They always work with a medical office for backup in case a medical situation arises.

At dermatologist's offices, they perform a similar role to the nurse practitioner at the gynecologist. They see patients for routine visits and checkups. If more challenging situations arise, the dermatologist sees the patient.

Some paramedical estheticians also have nursing degrees. Nurses can perform Botox and collagen injections, but paramedical estheticians can't in most states.

Some skin care clinics hire only nurses as paramedical estheticians. This ensures that the patient's medical skin care needs are addressed as they enjoy facials or light peels.

When working with a paramedical esthetician, you can get prescriptions for some skin care medications, such as Retin-A, Renova, and Differin, because a medical doctor oversees the clinic.

Wrinkle Guard

A phenol peel should only be done by a doctor in a doctor's office. If anyone other than a doctor offers to give you a phenol peel, run the other way. Fast. Also, it is unlikely that a nurse or esthetician would dispense Accutane because it's a dangerous, though effective drug that requires monthly blood work and close supervision by a doctor. Beware if an esthetician is dispensing Accutane.

Dermatologists

Skin doctors must have traditional medical training. They've been through medical school and have chosen skin as their specialty. They've done residency and internships at hospitals. They have years of experience under their belt before they ever set up a private practice.

Dermatologists usually have one of two specialties. The first is treating skin disorders, such as acne, eczema, and dermatitis. The second specialty is treating aging skin, such as doing Botox injections, Restylane injections, and laser treatments.

Dermatologists prescribe medications for everything you may need for your skin, both for cosmetic reasons, like wrinkles and sun damage, and for the health of your skin, such as psoriasis treatments. Dermatologists remove skin cancers and skin growths. They can work with lasers to remove spider veins and help smooth your face.

Skin-spiration

If you have a skin care concern that your esthetician can't resolve, set an appointment with a dermatologist. A good esthetician will refer you to a dermatologist when she can't be of help.

Whenever something unusual is going on with your skin, go to the dermatologist. By this we mean such things as odd discolorations, bumps, red spots, and itchy patches. If you suspect you have skin cancer, set an appointment that day. Never delay an appointment if you suspect you have skin cancer.

Dermatologists can inject Botox and collagen and can perform other skin-enhancing treatments.

Plastic Surgeons

Any medical doctor can call himself or herself a plastic surgeon. We think of a plastic surgeon as doing face-lifts, but any doctor could perform a face-lift. The designation isn't a clear medical specialty, but there is a board certification for Plastic Surgery: Cosmetic and Reconstructive from the American Society of Plastic Surgery-ASPS. This means you need to be very careful when choosing a plastic surgeon and only choose one who is board-certified by the ASPS.

Look for the designation "Board Certified by the American Board of Plastic Surgery" when you want some "work" done. These plastic surgeons are qualified to do partial or full face-lifts.

Procedures like eye lifts, cheek lifts, chin implants, cheekbone implants, forehead lifts, and more are all performed by plastic surgeons. They work in hospitals and in surgical centers specializing in outpatient procedures.

Plastic surgeons also do in-office procedures such as Botox injections, skin resurfacing, glycolic peels, laser skin resurfacing, and acne scar treatment.

You'll learn more about plastic surgery and how to choose a surgeon in Chapter 30.

> **Wrinkle Guard**
>
> Be sure to ask around for the best plastic surgeons in your area. Ask friends, dermatologists, skin care specialists, and even your hair stylist. Go the ASPS website at www.plastic-surgery.org to certified plastic surgeons in your area. Hair stylists see the scars and know who does good work and which plastic surgeons are sloppy.

The Least You Need to Know

- Makeup artists and permanent makeup artists are the only skin care professionals not licensed by the states.

- Skin care professionals take many hours of specialized training and pass state board exams before being licensed.

- Choose skin care professionals based on their experience and your skin care needs.

- The term "plastic surgeon" doesn't designate a medical specialty, so shop carefully before you have "work" done.

Chapter 28

Salon and Spa Treatments

In This Chapter

- ◆ The benefits of facial treatments
- ◆ De-stressing at the salon or spa
- ◆ Choosing a facial based on your skin type
- ◆ Correcting skin conditions with facials

For some people, a salon or spa facial seems like a totally self-indulgent luxury. Others consider them a necessity. In fact, you can achieve better skin without ever setting foot into a salon or spa, but a good facial can definitely go a long way in helping you meet your goal of clear, beautiful skin.

Studies show that facials lower your body's levels of the stress hormone, cortisol. This automatically reduces inflammation and soothes premature aging. During a facial, your face is pampered, cleansed, moisturized, peeled, and nourished, while your shoulders, face, or both are soothingly massaged. All of these procedures certainly benefit your skin.

In this chapter, you'll learn all about facials and what good they can do for your skin and your state of mind.

Facials as Pampering

Facials can be viewed in two ways. The first, and the primary focus of this chapter, is as treatment for your skin. Facials renew, rejuvenate, nourish, and heal your skin. The methods and treatments used are specifically designed with the science of skin care in mind.

The second and also very important part of facials is the relaxation quality. Few people today have time for self-pampering, and the pampering they do get is often mixed in with meeting other's needs—those of spouses, children, and employers.

A facial is your time just for you. You aren't even required to talk. You can just lie down and bliss out for an hour as someone else waits on you.

Researchers conducted a study on the relaxation qualities of facials. First, they measured the cortisol levels of a group of people by testing their saliva. Part of the group rested on the sofa for an hour. The rest of the group each received a personalized one-hour facial. After an hour, the sofa group had little to no reduction in cortisol levels. Those who relaxed with a facial did indeed relax—their cortisol levels were substantially reduced.

> **Skin-spiration**
>
> A facial is a time for relaxing. Check out the environment to make sure it meets your needs. Is the facial room quiet, private, and soothing? Is the music relaxing and nurturing? Do you like the skin care specialist? If not, shop around until you find an environment that appeals to you.

Pampering is important. It does far more for your well-being than you might think. Facials reduce your body's internal stress levels, which is vital for your health. High cortisol levels are associated with the onset of diabetes, high-blood pressure, heart disease, depression, anxiety, and autoimmune diseases.

The bottom line is this: Facials are good for your skin and your whole body. So go ahead and enjoy every second of pampering—it's more than self-indulgence, it's good for your skin and your health.

The Basic Components

Reading through a list of facial offerings at a salon or spa can be confusing. There are literally thousands of different types of facials. You'll find rejuvenating, purifying, balancing, oxygen, European, deep cleansing, alpha-beta peels, and many more. To tell you the truth, it's sometimes confusing to know what to ask for.

Fortunately, a good skin care technician knows what you need. No, not just by looking, but by asking you the right questions. Hopefully, at the salon or spa you've chosen, you are asked to fill out a questionnaire about your skin and your goals for your skin and for your facial. By knowing your skin type and any preexisting skin conditions, the technician can custom-tailor a facial to meet your needs.

For all of the thousands of specialized facials available, there are really only a handful of functions of a facial, which can be met singly or in combination. Those functions are:

◆ Moisturizing and hydrating. Facials add moisture to the surface of the skin by methods such as steam, humectants, occlusive masks, and hydrating creams.

◆ Cleansing. Facials use extraction to remove blackheads, whiteheads, and pimples. Cleansing can also include use of clay masks.

◆ Deep cleansing. Expect a deep-cleansing facial to include extractions. The skin care technician uses gloves, a magnification lens, and a needle. Before extractions, he or she softens the skin in preparation. Skin care technicians do extractions hygienically and correctly, so there's no danger of spreading or exacerbating the blemish. They also know when to leave a blemish alone.

◆ Peels. Exfoliation methods include enzymes, scrubs, and chemicals, such as glycolic, lactic, and salicylic acids. Many also include electric brushes.

◆ Microdermabrasion. The use of a microdermabrasion machine can be incorporated to remove dead skin cells from the face by having mineral crystals flow over the skin with a vacuum-type wand.

◆ Firming. Facials can use masks and other products that tighten and firm skin. This is great for aging skin.

◆ Nourishing. A facial may add nourishing ingredients, such as vitamins, minerals, and antioxidants, onto the skin.

◆ Lightening. Some facials use skin lighteners, such as licorice or weak solutions of hydroquinone.

◆ Massage. Many facials incorporate facial massage, but they can also include hand or shoulder massages.

Skin-spiration

Be sure to ask your skin care technician to customize your facial based on your skin's needs that day. Facials don't come in "one-size-fits-all" packages. Know your goal when you set your appointment.

Facials at salons and spas can include everything except medical treatments, such as heavy phenol peels, Botox, and collagen injections. Those are done only in medical offices.

A Facial Suited to Your Skin Type

Receiving the best facial means that the skin care technician knows your skin type. Each skin type requires specifically tailored treatments. The following recommendations are for skin that isn't affected by a more serious skin condition. Use the following only if your skin is functioning well at the time of the appointment:

◆ Normal skin can benefit from any type of facial, based on the skin's needs that day. The latest facial fad usually works as well as the tried-and-true basic moisturizing and cleansing facial.

◆ Oily skin requires deep cleansing. Enzymatic peels are good, as are salicylic acid peels. Microdermabrasion is fine, but there's a slight chance that it could over-stimulate oil production or lead to breakouts and congestion. Clay masks are recommended for deep cleansing and for reducing the amount of oil on the surface of the skin.

◆ The rule of thumb for sensitive skin is that less is best. Treatments can include a small amount of steam, acupressure massage, or lymphatic drainage. A cooling mask that doesn't dry on the skin is quite soothing, but avoid the heavy creams, which can be irritating.

Wrinkle Guard

Don't schedule a facial right before a major event, such as a wedding, photo shoot, or video taping session. If your skin becomes irritated or inflamed following the facial, you won't have time for it to calm down and heal. No one wants to be a red-faced bride.

◆ Oil-dry skin needs hydration and stimulation to aid the skin in producing more oil. Using treatments like a paraffin mask, a glycolic peel, microdermabrasion, steam, and intense creams can be beneficial.

◆ Acne-type skin needs to be calmed and soothed with deep cleansing and perhaps a salicylic exfoliation. Avoid a facial massage, as it can be too stimulating for your skin, but a shoulder or hand massage is great. Acne skin needs extractions along with other deep-cleansing treatments, such as clay masks and salicylic peels.

Don't expect your skin care technician to use all of these techniques at each facial. Most likely, he or she will give your skin the treatments that best fit your immediate needs.

Facials for Skin Conditions

A good time to schedule a facial is when you're experiencing temporary skin conditions, such as congestion or breakout. In fact, it's great to schedule facials every month for your skin, regardless of its condition. Inform your skin care specialist of your needs, because the standard facial for your skin type needs to be modified to help correct your condition. Temporary skin conditions are discussed in detail in Part 4 of this book.

A good skin care technician knows how to help you solve temporary skin conditions. Ask your skin care technician to advise you about special skin treatments you can do at home to continue the healing effects of the facial. You may want to schedule a full series of salon or spa facials to correct skin conditions such as ...

> **Skin-spiration**
>
> A great time for a revitalizing facial is after a vacation, airplane travel, or completing a stressful work deadline. Use the facial to rebalance your skin and replenish nutrients and moisture.

- Congestion and breakouts. Your facial goal is extraction and removal of dead skin cells so your skin is clear. You need a deep-cleansing facial with exfoliation. Salicylic acid or a clay mask will work well for exfoliation, and perhaps your skin care technician will use both. A steam treatment will get the blood flowing to your skin. This helps it heal more quickly. Extraction of blackheads, whiteheads, and pimples will clear up some of the congestion. Microdermabrasion can also work well.

- Rosacea. Your facial goal is calming and soothing. Your skin needs to be treated very gently. Make sure the skin care technician is aware of the rosacea and doesn't over-stimulate your skin. Think calm and cool. Avoid electrical brushes and microdermabrasion. Cold stone treatments for the face are excellent, as are cooling masks, a shoulder massage, and a very gentle peel, preferably with an enzyme or with lactic acid. The relaxation aspect of your facial helps to reduce inflammation and irritation. For information on cold-stone treatments, see Chapter 13.

- Dehydration. Your goal is to add moisture back into your skin. Steaming is good, as is a facial massage with moisturizing products. Peel with either an enzyme peel or glycolic acid. Paraffin masks are an excellent way to infuse moisture. Microdermabrasion can polish the skin and provide a gentle exfoliation treatment. Finish up with humectants and moisturizers.

◆ Sensitized skin. Talk with the skin care technician to determine the root cause of your skin condition. Your goal is to calm and soothe the skin and to relax. Your skin needs gentle treatments, such as a cooling mask, shoulder massage, and lymphatic massage. Extraction is fine if your skin needs it. If your skin is sensitized as a result of illness, antibiotics, or chemotherapy, use clay masks or green tea compresses to draw toxins out of the skin.

◆ Sun damage. Your goal is to reduce sun damage and increase cell turnover rate. Peel with microdermabrasion, glycolic acid, or a combination of AHAs and BHAs. The skin care technician can be more aggressive with your skin and could possibly do two peels because of the high keratinization levels of your skin. First do a BHA peel and then a glycolic peel. Steam is beneficial, as are humectants and moisturizing creams.

◆ Pigmentation. Your goal is to have your darker pigmentation areas appear lighter, along with receiving a facial to suit your skin type. One or even two peels with microdermabrasion, glycolic acid, or a combination of AHAs and BHAs to increase cell turnover rate can help. Use bleaching herbals, such as red raspberry and licorice. A mild hydroquinone cream is also effective. Your skin care technician might suggest that you consult with a dermatologist to inquire about a prescription for a high-percentage hydroquinone cream or Retin-A. If your pigmentation is caused by illness, then your skin type determines your facial treatments.

Wrinkle Guard

If your skin care technician uses glycolic or salicylic peels on your skin, you can receive more benefit from your facial by using exfoliating products with AHAs and BHAS regularly as part of your home skin care ritual.

◆ Premature aging. Your goal is to reduce the appearance of aging. The skin care technician can stimulate the skin with vitamin C and other nourishing ingredients, such as essential fatty acids, vitamins, and minerals. Your skin needs stimulation to increase cell turnover rate. Peel with glycolic or lactic acid or feed skin with oxygen. An energetic massage helps to increase blood circulation to the skin. Talk with your skin care technician about the causes of your prematurely aging skin so that you can make lifestyle changes to correct the condition.

◆ Menopausal skin. Your goal is to firm, tighten, and stimulate skin to increase cell turnover rate. Apply phytoestrogen products directly on skin to help plump it up. Use stronger glycolic peels at 30 to 40 percent solution and a pH of 2.5 to 3. Microdermabrasion can also be helpful. Apply moisturizing products.

Schedule a facial when you want to be pampered, when your skin is acting up, and about a week before a big event. You should also consider having a facial with the change of seasons for seasonal cleansing. Think of it as spring cleaning for the skin.

The Least You Need to Know

◆ Facials are excellent for getting your skin in great shape and for maintaining great skin.

◆ Facials reduce cortisol stress levels at the same time that they soothe skin inflammation and irritation due to stress.

◆ Ask for a facial that's best for your genetic skin type.

◆ Inform your skin care technician if you have a skin condition that requires special attention.

Chapter 29

Medical and Paramedical Treatments

In This Chapter

- ◆ Learning about wrinkle fillers and skin plumpers
- ◆ Noninvasive face-lift techniques
- ◆ Understanding Botox
- ◆ Lessening the appearance of acne scars
- ◆ Avoiding outdated procedures

Medical procedures for the skin that don't require full-blown surgery are becoming increasingly popular. Both men and women can have wrinkles soothed, skin resurfaced, broken capillaries removed, and lips plumped without going "under the knife." Set an appointment at the doctor's office and you can usually be in and out within an hour.

You may be able to go right back to work, or you may need to take a week or so off for recovery time. Either way, your face and skin will look younger and you'll enjoy the freshness you see when you look in the mirror. Of course, all procedures have some risk associated with them.

In this chapter, you'll learn about medical treatments ranging from Botox to laser resurfacing. You'll know what each treatment can and can't do, the standard recovery times, and how long each treatment lasts.

Is It Time?

There's no set formula for when you may want to consider medical skin treatments. Perhaps you've wanted your acne scars minimized for years. Perhaps those furrow lines between your brows all of a sudden seem to make you appear unhappy or angry.

> **CAUTION**
>
> **Wrinkle Guard**
>
> All medical skin care procedures can be overdone. You've undoubtedly seen photos of celebrities with overly puffy lips from too much collagen or totally expressionless faces filled with too much muscle-paralyzing Botox. Don't get carried away with these procedures. Only do what it takes to achieve a rested, relaxed, and youthful face without looking ridiculous.

The truth is, you'll know. And when you do, it's time to consider finding a doctor who does skin treatments at the office. You may be treated by the doctor directly or by a trained paramedical esthetician or nurse. Just be sure that you are being treated in a medical facility that has a doctor who oversees all procedures. Medical insurance doesn't cover these types of cosmetic procedures, so you don't want to take risks with your care.

The best way to find a doctor is to ask around. Ask friends, skin care specialists, your dermatologist, your family-care physician, and even your hair stylist. Look for a doctor that you'll feel comfortable calling on for additional procedures in the future.

Collagen

Collagen injections take mere moments to perform but can take years from your face. Collagen is a natural protein that provides texture, resilience, and shape to your skin and face. The collagen used for facial injections comes from human tissue as well as bovine (cow) tissue. Injectable collagen is used to replace lost skin tissue and to fill in depressions and wrinkles.

Before you undertake collagen injections, you need to have two skin tests in a one-month period, two weeks apart, to make sure you aren't allergic to the substance used. Allergic reactions occur in only 2 percent of the people who receive injections. Collagen is considered safe by the FDA.

Injected collagen fills in scars, including acne scars and scars from injuries. Injected into lips, collagen makes them thicker and more luscious and youthful looking. It's also used to fill in any kind of wrinkle around the mouth, eyes, and chin. It isn't recommended for depressions with sharp edges and narrow acne scars.

Collagen does dissipate into the body over time. It's impossible to tell how long your collagen injections will last, but the time range is anywhere from 90 days to as long as eight months, depending on how fast your body metabolizes. The faster it metabolizes, the less time the collagen injection will last.

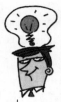

Skin-spiration

The durability of collagen or Restylane injections is related to the location of the injection. Lips absorb the substance more quickly than acne scars on the sides of the face.

The shots are sometimes painful, but the pain lasts only a very short time. It takes about a week for the collagen to settle into the right place in the skin. Don't schedule a fancy date that night or a big business presentation for the next day. Your face could be red and inflamed following the procedure, and this can last up to a week.

After the collagen settles, it can look smooth on the surface of your skin, but it could feel bumpy to the touch.

The price of collagen injections varies with the doctor. You are usually charged by the amount of collagen injected in cubic centimeters (cc's). Seldom will the doctor give you a set cost ahead of time, as it's impossible to know how much collagen you'll need.

To soothe your skin after a collagen injection, calm it down with ice for the first 24 hours. Avoid using other products as the small holes from the injection could let bacteria enter your skin and cause an infection.

There are reported cases of people developing an autoimmune disease after collagen injections, but at this time scientists haven't proven that the injections caused the diseases. Weigh your interest in the procedure carefully. Before you sign on for collagen injections, check out the newest wrinkle filler, Restylane, discussed in the section that follows.

Restylane

The FDA (Food and Drug Administration) recently approved Restylane for injection to correct moderate to severe facial folds and wrinkles. It's made from biodegradable, nonanimal, and stabilized hyaluronic acid, which is found in human skin tissue. Hyaluronic acid naturally provides volume and fullness to the skin. It can hold 1,000 times its weight in water, but its presence decreases as a person ages.

Restylane restores the youthful, plump appearance of the skin. In a sense, it restores the function of natural hyaluronic acid, if only temporarily. The results last a couple months longer than collagen. You can expect a Restylane injection to last between 6 and 12 months.

Restylane is an improvement over collagen, which is typically made from bovine sources. It has none of the complications associated with collagen, such as allergic reactions, so you don't need a skin patch test prior to injection. Patients treated with Restylane reported less bruising, swelling, pain, and tenderness than with collagen injections.

In addition to smoothing out wrinkles, Restylane is used to increase the fullness of the lips. Expect a day or two of redness and swelling after Restylane injections.

Because Restylane causes fewer complications than collagen, it's predicted that Restylane will replace collagen as the wrinkle filler of choice. You pay by the cubic centimeter, the same as with collagen, but the total injection volume needed to produce optimal results with Restylane is usually less than with collagen. However, you can expect to about pay about the same amount for both types of treatment.

Botox

Botox injections are seemingly a miracle for erasing furrows between the eyebrows and the nasal labial folds between the nose and corners of the mouth. Botox is purified botulinum bacteria. This is the same bacteria that causes a severe and often fatal form of food poisoning. The difference is that the botulinum bacteria in Botox are a purified form that won't cause illness. It simply paralyzes certain muscles of the face.

Botox works well for forehead furrows, crow's feet, and frown lines. The results last for four to six months. You pay by the number of units of Botox injected into your face. Sometimes an injection doesn't take and you'll need a touch-up. One in 10 people develop bruising from the injection, and the injections are sometimes painful.

Skin-spiration

If you choose to have Botox injections, you could find that over time you break the habit of contracting the muscles in your face that cause wrinkles and expressions lines.

Temporary side effects include drooping of the eyebrows or eyelids that lasts three to six months, but is always reversible. Drooping is rare when the injection is done by a qualified person. Double vision has been reported, but the incidence is rare. The condition lasts from three to six months and is also reversible. There are no known long-term side effects.

Don't use Botox if you have myasthenia gravis, a neuromuscular disease such as neuropathy or muscular dystrophy, or an allergy to human albumin or botulinum toxin. You can't use Botox injections if you are pregnant or breastfeeding, have had an alcoholic beverage within seven days, or have taken aspirin or an anti-inflammatory medication within 14 days.

After an injection, you can't lie down for four hours. Be careful not to massage the treated muscles, because the Botox can spread to the muscles around the eye area. You need to exercise the injected muscles every 15 minutes for an hour after treatment because Botox attaches best to active muscles. You can repeat Botox treatments every four to six months.

Botox seems like a miracle, but before you schedule an appointment, determine how much expression you want to retain in your face. Figure out what works for you and your lifestyle. It's wonderful to erase furrows, but a face void of any expression can appear boring and uninterested to others.

Thermal Lift

Imagine getting a face-lift without surgery, scars, or any recovery time. Seem like a fantasy? Not for some people who can benefit from thermal lift procedures. Thermal lifts give you many of the benefits of a surgical face-lift as well as renewing the texture of your skin by creating new and denser collagen, causing an appreciable increase in the thickness of your skin. With a thermal lift, there are no needles and no injections into your skin. How can this be? Using radio-frequency (RF) energy, sometimes known by its trade name, Thermage.

The catch is that only some people can benefit from Thermage and often the people who have the most skin to tighten are least likely to respond to the treatment. But if it works, it's wonderful. You can contact a dermatologist or plastic surgeon who uses Thermage and ask for a free consultation to determine if you're a good candidate. Yes, they do turn some candidates away.

Radio-frequency energy reduces the signs of skin aging by tightening tissue. The radio-frequency energy uniformly heats the dermis while cooling and protecting the epidermis. The collagen in the skin contracts and new collagen is produced over time. You'll see results appear gradually over two to six months and possibly sooner.

On average, the results last up to two years, sometimes longer depending on the rate at which your skin is aging. You can reduce the rate at which your skin ages by following the recommendations in Part 5 of this book.

The actual process is somewhat uncomfortable, so an anesthetic, or numbing cream, is applied about an hour before the procedure begins. From start to finish, a full-face treatment takes about three hours. The good news is, you'll leave the doctor's office with some redness, but you can go right back to work. There's no downtime. However, you may not want to plan a big night out later that evening.

Laser Resurfacing

Consider this treatment only if you have severe wrinkling, significant abnormal pigmentation, or deep acne scars. Laser resurfacing is a medical procedure that's invasive and requires downtime for healing. As it resurfaces the skin, the laser burns away outer layers. This triggers the fibroblasts that produce collagen to replace what's been burned off.

Laser resurfacing is excellent for reducing fine lines, cross-hatched lines, and abnormal pigmentation. It can tighten fine lines around the mouth in smokers and whistlers. Lasers can repair broken capillaries and some acne scarring. It may not remove all acne pock marks, but can make them less visible. Laser resurfacing doesn't work for sagging skin. If that's your primary concern, you should consider a thermal lift or surgical face-lift.

Skin-spiration

No matter what procedure you've chosen, be gentle with yourself during the recovery phase. It simply takes time to heal. It might take you a longer time to heal than the average, or you may heal faster. There's no way to know in advance. Stay in touch with your doctor to make sure you are healing well. Avoid getting nervous and upset, because these emotions can actually lengthen your healing time.

Because laser resurfacing is invasive, it puts your skin into repair mode. It invokes the entire inflammation system, as you get somewhere between a first-degree and second-degree burn. Estimate your recovery time at three weeks, and you'll need to hide out for a while as your face heals. You'll be put on a round of antibiotics to prevent infection, and you'll need pain pills during the healing process. Usually a person requires several laser resurfacing sessions to achieve the desired results.

Possible side effects include scarring from the burns and an increase in abnormal pigmentation. Before you schedule a laser resurfacing treatment, be sure that your doctor is highly experienced with laser and that he or she doesn't have a heavy hand. It's less risky to have several sessions than to have too much done in one session, as there's more possibility of undesirable side effects.

Before you sign up for laser resurfacing, check out the photorejuvenation systems in the next section. Perhaps you can achieve excellent results without resorting to an invasive procedure.

Photorejuvenation Systems

Also known as Foto-Facial Rejuvenation with Intense Pulsed Light (IPL), this procedure is noninvasive and can correct skin concerns such as pigmentation, age spots, very fine lines, sun damage, and can improve skin texture. But that's not all. It can reduce the appearance of rosacea, spider veins, birthmarks, and sun damage, plus help heal acne. After the procedure, your skin will feel smoother and look more evenly toned.

Skin-spiration

When you're considering a medical skin procedure, do your research on the Internet. You can find answers to your questions, known side effects, and even comments from others about the success of their procedures.

There's no anticipated downtime following a photorejuvenation treatment, but you could experience redness and irritation for several hours. Don't plan a big event for a couple of days following your treatment. Some people can apply some makeup immediately following a treatment and return to work. The results appear gradually, so you'll most likely require about five treatments in all. Each treatment takes about 30 to 45 minutes. The machine is passed over the skin and the procedure takes about an hour. Your skin shouldn't hurt, but it could tingle.

The treatment is safe, but limit your sun exposure afterward. In fact, you should always limit sun exposure and be sure to wear a sunscreen.

Photorejuvenation doesn't work to eliminate or lessen acne scars. If that is your primary concern, you should consider laser resurfacing.

High-Powered Microdermabrasion

Similar to microdermabrasion performed by a skin-care specialist, but used only by a qualified medical person because of its intensity and depth of treatment, high-powered microdermabrasion removes dead skin cells and helps improve the appearance of fine lines, and abnormal pigmentations.

Wrinkle Guard

Sometimes microdermabrasion is recommended to reduce broken capillaries. It won't do this and can sometimes make broken capillaries worse. Instead, consider using laser resurfacing for broken capillaries.

For the treatment, you lie down while the esthetician passes a wand over the surface of your skin. The wand sweeps mineral crystals across your face. Each session lasts about 45 minutes. Microdermabrasion is definitely less invasive than laser resurfacing and this treatment is great for maintaining the results of laser resurfacing. It's also excellent as a medical facial. Your recovery time is usually one night or one full day.

Other Treatments

These treatments are used less frequently than the ones listed in the previous sections. They are less popular either because they have undesirable side effects or because they have been supplanted by other easier and less invasive techniques.

Other treatments include:

- Fat injections or liposculpture. Used for the same purpose as collagen and Restylane. Fat is harvested from the patient's own unwanted fat stores, then injected into the face to plump up lips or cheeks or to treat deep folds. The procedure takes more time than the other procedures, and if a person gains weight, the injected areas can gain weight, too.

- Dermabrasion. A highly invasive procedure that goes far beyond microdermabrasion and is more intense than laser resurfacing. The epidermis is literally sanded off the entire face. You come out looking like raw hamburger. It's a very heavy-duty experience, and you'll wind up with open wounds and require heavy doses of antibiotics. It sounds agonizing, and it is. This procedure is seldom used today.

- Phenol peels. The strongest chemical peel available uses carbolic acid. Essentially, it burns off many layers of the skin, and is very painful. It takes three weeks to heal and requires rounds of antibiotics to prevent infections.

CAUTION

Wrinkle Guard

When selecting a medical skin care doctor, make sure the practitioner is up-to-date on and experienced with the least invasive methods for correcting your skin condition. Usually, the less invasive the better.

If a medical specialist recommends one of these treatments, ask if other, less invasive treatments with fewer side effects would work for you. Sometimes discomfort is the price of gaining better skin, but the least discomfort is always best and safest.

The Least You Need to Know

◆ Many excellent noninvasive skin treatments are effective in correcting skin conditions.

◆ Use laser resurfacing to lessen the appearance of acne scars.

◆ Botox works to paralyze muscles that cause furrows and wrinkles.

◆ Restylane is quickly replacing collagen for filling skin lines and folds.

◆ Avoid outdated medical skin treatments, such as phenol peels, dermabrasion, and fat injections.

Chapter 30

Plastic Surgery

In This Chapter

- Finding a plastic surgeon
- Evaluating your plastic surgery needs
- The right time for plastic surgery
- Procedures and recovery
- Expectations and lasting results

It seems like it's on everyone's lips these days. Plastic surgery is more popular than ever, with television reality shows and magazines promoting "Extreme Makeovers," friends and relatives praising its benefits, and the continued pastime of guessing which celebrity has had it.

Cosmetic plastic surgery is the term for surgical procedures used to enhance appearance. One day you may see your reflection and wonder just who that is staring back at you. Perhaps your eyes look tired all the time, or you have frown lines that won't go away. Thousands of people each year have plastic surgery to help them feel good about the way they look.

In this chapter, we'll tell you all about the different kinds of cosmetic surgical procedures and how they're used to enhance appearance. Whether it's just a brow lift or a full face-lift, plastic surgery may offer the improvement you're looking for.

The Surgeon Makes the Difference

It probably goes without saying that you don't choose a plastic surgeon like you would a plumber, picking the cheapest and most convenient name out of the phone book. After all, this is surgery for your face we're talking about, and unlike makeup, the results of plastic surgery cannot be washed away. So be smart and cautious in your selection.

Skin-spiration

Plastic surgery isn't just for women. More and more, men are deciding to have cosmetic surgical procedures to enhance their looks and to maintain their appearance for professional advantage.

Here are a few ways to select a surgeon:

◆ Choose a plastic surgeon based on a reference from a friend or relative who has had surgery with great results.

◆ Ask your primary care physician for a referral.

◆ Call the American Board of Plastic Surgeons and get a referral for surgeons in your area. Phone them at 215-587-9322 or visit www.abplsurg.org.

Interview two or three different surgeons before making your decision. Ask to see photos of their before and after results. You want to feel comfortable with the surgeon and his or her staff, and you'll want their opinions of which procedures you need. Most importantly, you want to make sure that the surgeon is a *board-certified plastic surgeon* and that the surgical facility is accredited and licensed by the state where it is located. You can check the facility's accreditation status by calling the American Association for Accreditation of Ambulatory Surgery Facilities (AAAASF) at 1-800-545-5222 (www.aaaasf.org).

It's never recommended to use a surgeon who isn't board certified! You wouldn't let your cable guy color your hair, would you? Well, you can redye your hair, but plastic surgery is permanent.

Clarifying Words

Board-certified physicians are surgeons certified by the American Board of Plastic Surgery (ABPS). They must undergo rigorous training, including medical school, a plastic surgery residency program, and an additional minimum of five years of surgical training. A surgeon must also pass comprehensive oral and written exams in order to be ABPS-certified. The ABPS is the only board recognized to certify surgeons in plastic surgery of the face and body by the American Board of Medical Specialties.

From Eye-Lifts to Face-Lifts

When most of us hear about cosmetic plastic surgery, we think face-lift. You might consider a face-lift if you have deep wrinkles, sagging cheekbones, loss of definition in the jaw line, deep lines from the nose to the mouth, and/or wrinkles, sagging, or excess fatty tissue in the neck. A face-lift can improve the sagging and wrinkling that comes with age and leave you with a firmer and refreshed appearance.

But you may not require an entire face-lift. If your eyes always look tired or droopy, or you have bags underneath them, cosmetic eyelid surgery may be all you need. Cosmetic eyelid surgery can improve the appearance of the upper and lower eyelids, helping you look brighter, rested, and more refreshed.

A forehead lift, or brow lift, may be the right procedure for you if you have deep frown lines, sagging eyebrows, a low brow line, deep horizontal creases on the forehead, or furrows between the eyebrows and nose. Like cosmetic eyelid surgery, a forehead lift can improve your appearance by making you look more youthful and alert.

Facial implants are used to improve the contour of the face and provide proportion. There are a variety of implants available for the chin, jaw, and cheek. Facial implants can greatly enhance facial features by providing an aesthetically pleasing profile and conformity of size and shape.

Cosmetic surgery of the nose, officially known as rhinoplasty but more frequently referred to as a "nose job," is the most common procedure performed on young adults. If your nose seems out of proportion to your other facial features, is crooked or off-center, seems too large or wide, or if the tip droops or is thick, then you might consider rhinoplasty to correct the situation.

> **Body of Knowledge**
>
> Multiple plastic surgeries are often performed simultaneously to provide the best results. Sometimes facial implants are inserted at the same time as a face-lift, or cosmetic eye surgery and a forehead lift are done together. Your surgeon will discuss with you the best procedure or procedures necessary to achieve the desired outcome.

Is This Your Time?

When is the "right" time to consider plastic surgery? If you look older than you feel, if people always ask you if you're angry, or if you look like you need a nap, maybe the time is right. And it's not just age that impacts our appearance. Heredity, environmental factors, stress, and more also contribute. Although a young adult may not require a face-lift, he or she may need a forehead lift to raise a low brow line. And while most face-lifts are performed on 40- to 60-year-olds, perfectly good results can be achieved for a 70-year-old.

Cosmetic surgical procedures can enhance your appearance at any age—within reason, of course. It's more common for young adults to have rhinoplasty or facial implants to improve the contour of the face, but surgeons recommend that facial growth is complete before having this type of procedure. For girls that would be about age 13 or 14, and for boys it would be 14 or 15. The surgery should be the teenager's idea, obviously, and should be approved and endorsed by both the parents and physician.

> **Body of Knowledge**
>
> About 44 percent of all plastic surgeries are performed on adults age 35 to 40. The next largest group is the 19- to 34-year-olds at 25 percent. Those aged 51 to 64 make up 23 percent, and those older than age 65 account for the rest (8 percent).

Face-lifts and forehead lifts are more popular for 40- to 60-year-olds, while cosmetic eye surgery is popular for those in their 30s and older. There are no firm guidelines, however, and your age does not always determine your appearance. There are some people who look much older than they are, and would simply rather that their appearance match their age.

Age is not the only issue to think about when considering plastic surgery. Your overall health is important, as is your state of mind. There are certain things you must discuss with your surgeon. These should be covered during your consultation.

Health Issues

Your physical health will be assessed. Beyond your regular health history, your surgeon will also want to know about any previous surgeries, medical conditions, and treatments you may have received.

Full disclosure increases your chances for successful surgery. In some situations, the surgeon may decline to operate based on a person's health profile.

Medications

You must tell your surgeon about all medications you are taking. This includes vitamins and herbal supplements. Your surgeon may recommend that you stop taking some supplements and over-the-counter medications a couple of weeks before surgery, as they could interfere with your healing or anesthetic. Be sure to follow his or her recommendations.

Weight

If you are overweight and plan on losing 15 pounds or more, tell your surgeon, because the results of your surgery may be affected. Some surgeons may recommend that you lose weight before they perform a facial procedure, so that you get the best results.

Medical Conditions

Certain medical conditions require that surgery be approached with extra caution. These include blood-clotting problems, high blood pressure, allergies, eye diseases, thyroid disorders, cardiovascular disease, circulatory disorders, and diabetes.

> **Body of Knowledge**
>
> If you are a smoker, your surgeon will ask you to stop smoking for a period of time before your surgery. This will assure a higher level of success. Smoking inhibits blood flow and it can impede the healing process. And, just think, this may be your golden opportunity to quit smoking forever.

What You Can Expect

Popular culture would lead us to believe that having plastic surgery will completely change your life for the better. If you'd just get a nip here and a tuck there, your love life would improve, you'd get that big promotion at work, and your social calendar would be full for the next 50 years. It would be great if all that happened, but it won't.

Plastic surgery doesn't work that way. What you can reasonably expect is to have fewer bags, wrinkles, and sags. This could very well make you appear more attractive and could improve your professional life, especially if you spend time with the public, as in a sales or media career.

Skin-spiration

Cosmetic plastic surgery can make your appearance more youthful and refreshed, and that in turn may enhance your confidence and self-esteem. Many people are using plastic surgery as a tool to become more competitive in the job market—and also in the adult dating game. Sales people, marketing representatives, and people who work under the scrutiny of the public eye find that plastic surgery pays.

However, although you can expect some positive results from cosmetic plastic surgery, it won't change your personality or your behaviors, or cure you of your bad habits. It won't make people love you more or improve a bad relationship. That's your responsibility. Before you have surgery, make sure you understand your personal expectations and discuss them with your surgeon.

If you are considering plastic surgery, there are some important factors to consider which will be covered in the sections that follow.

The Right Procedure for You

By the time you phone the surgeon's office, you need to know your appearance goals. Most likely, you'll already have something in mind. As you talk with your surgeon, he or she will advise you about the procedures best suited to your appearance goals.

Cost

The average U.S. costs are:

◆ Face-lift: $8,000

◆ Forehead lift: $4,000

◆ Eyelid surgery (upper and lower): $4,500

◆ Rhinoplasty: $5,000

◆ Chin or cheek implants: $3,500

These prices are averages. You'll find the prices vary based on your geographic location and from surgeon to surgeon.

Insurance seldom pays for plastic surgery, which means you'll be responsible for the full cost. Many surgeons now accept major credit cards. Some have time payment plans. Be sure to discuss fees and payments with your surgeon.

Most surgeons have a set fee for each surgery. This fee includes everything from the anesthesiologist to the recovery room. You'll know exactly what the total cost is before you schedule a procedure. This prevents any billing surprises later on down the road.

Safety and Risks

By choosing a surgeon certified by the American Board of Plastic Surgery and having your surgery done at an accredited and certified surgical facility, you are taking steps in assuring your safety. You must also be sure to follow your surgeon's instructions carefully. No surgery is without risk. Thousands of people undergo plastic surgery each year with no complications. But complications do occur. Make sure you understand the risks before you schedule your surgery.

Location: Hospital or Surgical Center

Depending on the procedure, your surgery will be performed in either an office-based surgical suite, an outpatient surgical center, or a hospital. Most surgeries are performed on an outpatient basis and you'll go home the same day. However, your doctor may want you to stay overnight at a hospital, depending on the extent of the surgery, the state of your overall health, and the doctor's personal preference.

Preparation

Your plastic surgeon will give you specific instructions for the days, and sometimes weeks, before your surgery. You may be asked to discontinue certain medications and stop smoking. Be sure to follow all of your surgeon's instructions for the best results.

Anesthesia

Your surgeon and the anesthesiologist work together to determine what kind of anesthesia you'll need. With general anesthesia, you'll be unconscious throughout the entire procedure. Sometimes, local anesthesia is used in combination with an intravenous sedative, so you will feel drowsy and relaxed. You may be aware of some tugging and mild discomfort.

> **Body of Knowledge**
>
> Even if your surgery is performed at an office-based or outpatient surgical facility, make sure your surgeon has operating privileges for your specific procedure at an accredited local hospital. This is for backup in case you need to be taken to a hospital. Ask the surgeon or call your local hospital for verification.

Duration of the Procedure

This depends on what procedures you're having done. Face-lifts take several hours, especially when performed with another procedure. Some surgeons may actually schedule two separate sessions. Facial implants, forehead lifts, and rhinoplasty take one to two hours, and eyelid surgery takes approximately one to three hours.

Post-Surgery Recovery

After your surgery is completed, you'll be taken to a recovery room where your vital signs will be closely monitored and you'll be given medication to control any pain or

Wrinkle Guard

The prices for surgery can vary widely from surgeon to surgeon. As you shop around, you may find that the price of a procedure can vary from $5,500 to $20,000. Choose your surgeon based on skill, not necessarily price. Ask the high-priced surgeon why his or her rates are so much higher than those of others.

discomfort. You'll probably have bandages to control swelling and, if you've had a face-lift, there may be small drainage tubes placed beneath the skin.

If you've had rhinoplasty you'll likely have a splint on the bridge of the nose to hold the tissues in place and packing inside the nostrils. Cold compresses and lubricating ointment may be applied to your eyes after eyelid surgery, and you may have loose gauze covering your eyes.

If you're not staying overnight, you'll be able to go home a few hours after surgery. For your safety, be sure to ask a friend to stay with you the first night after surgery. Before you leave, you'll receive specific instructions for recovering at home.

Home Recovery Time

You're home, possibly bandaged, and feeling somewhat bruised and swollen. Now what? You certainly don't look like the "glorious new you" you were expecting. Not yet, at least. Patience. A little time and healing and you'll be back to your old self. Better than your old self, in fact.

Follow your surgeon's instructions. Do exactly what your post-op information sheet tells you to do. If something doesn't seem right, phone the surgeon's office immediately. Otherwise, relax and give yourself time to heal. Take your medications as advised.

When do you get back to normal? Individual recovery times vary, but there are some general "stepping stones" you can expect while on your way to recovery.

For the first few days you will definitely want to take it easy. Your surgeon may instruct you to keep your head elevated, even when you sleep, and avoid any strenuous activity. Keep in mind, you've just had surgery, so plan on some swelling, bruising, discomfort, and tightness, but this will be temporary.

In addition to the common side effects and expectations, here are some rules of thumb for each type of procedure.

Face-Lift

Your skin will be tender, tight, bruised, and perhaps numb. Swelling peaks during the first week, then lessens in the following weeks. You'll have your bandages removed sometime during the first week. Your stitches will be removed, or they may be the kind that dissolve naturally.

Most bruising, if any, disappears within two to three weeks, and by that time you'll be back to most of your normal activities. Go slow on exercise and anything strenuous. Expect to be back at work within one to two weeks.

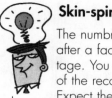

Skin-spiration

The numbness in your face after a face-lift is an advantage. You won't feel some of the recovery pain. Expect the numbness to dissipate over a couple of months.

Wear sunglasses for a week or two when you need to shop at the grocery store. Change your hairstyle at least slightly before you expect to encounter friends. That way they're more likely to comment on your hair than ask if you had "some work done."

Forehead Lift

In addition to the expected swelling and bruising, you may have numbness and headaches. Take it easy for the first couple of days. You may resume light activity as soon as you feel ready, but you may need to avoid strenuous activity for several weeks. Your bruising should subside within two to three weeks. You should be able return to work within 7 to 10 days, even sooner if you had an endoscopic procedure.

Eyelid Surgery

In addition to swelling and bruising, you may experience a tightness of the eyelids, dry eyes, and possibly itching and burning. These symptoms can be controlled with ointments, cold compresses, and medication. You may resume light activity after a few days, and may return to work after 7 to 10 days.

You can read again after two or three days, and if you wear contacts, use them after two weeks or so with your surgeon's permission. You should avoid strenuous activities for about three weeks. Your stitches, if you have them, will be removed after 5 to 10 days.

You may wear makeup, and it is recommended that you wear dark glasses to protect your eyes.

Rhinoplasty

Your beautiful new nose won't make its final appearance for a while. Bruising and swelling around the eyes and nose is to be expected, and you may experience some

Wrinkle Guard

Protecting your skin from exposure to the sun always makes sense, but it is crucial after plastic surgery. Limit exposure to direct sunlight, and always wear sun block when outdoors.

stiffness and bleeding. The swelling peaks within 10 days and then subsides. Your stitches and packing will be removed and you'll discontinue using the splint within one to two weeks.

You may return to work and resume normal activities after one or two weeks and after several weeks you may return to more strenuous activities. Your new nose is sensitive, though, so avoid activities that could injure it. That means no dodgeball, for sure.

Facial Implants

Tenderness, swelling, bruising, and some numbness and stiffness are to be expected. You'll want to take it easy for the first few days and keep your head elevated. You may return to work after one week and you should have a normal appearance within two to four weeks. Be careful not to engage in any activity that could bump your face. Once again, no dodgeball.

Long-Lasting Results

Your recovery is complete. You're looking refreshed, rejuvenated, and relaxed. But just how long will it last? The answer depends on your procedure.

If you've had a face-lift and/or forehead lift, you can expect good results for at least 5 to 10 years. Eyelid surgery results can last for several years and, in some instances, can be permanent. The results of facial implants and rhinoplasty are permanent.

Wrinkle Guard

Don't become a plastic surgery addict. Yes, you want to look as refreshed, enhanced, and natural as possible. However, frequently repeated surgeries may leave your face looking tight and frighteningly unnatural.

Your surgeon will monitor your healing. It's important to be open with your plastic surgeon throughout the entire process. This will not only help your surgeon, it will also help you in your progress.

Now, when you are asked about your great new look, how will you respond? Great vacation? Or maybe you'll just hand over your plastic surgeon's card and smile.

The Least You Need to Know

♦ Select a plastic surgeon who is certified by the American Board of Plastic Surgery.

♦ Keep your expectations natural and realistic to avoid disappointment.

♦ Your plastic surgeon will help you decide which procedure is appropriate for your age and health.

♦ Recovery times vary depending on the procedure.

♦ Your results may last for years, and in some cases, such as rhinoplasty, are permanent.

Glossary

allantion   A derivative of uric acid that is soothing and calming to the skin. It's found in roots, bark, and grains, and is used in skin products for healing.

antioxidants   Chemicals that neutralize free radicals that cause damage to the body and skin. These come from eating fruits and vegetables and also can be applied topically to help heal the surface of the skin.

board-certified physicians   In relation to plastic surgery, surgeons who are certified by the American Board of Plastic Surgery (ABPS). They undergo rigorous training, including medical school, a plastic surgery residency program, and an additional minimum of five years of surgical training. A surgeon must also pass comprehensive oral and written exams in order to be ABPS certified. The ABPS is the only board recognized to certify surgeons in plastic surgery of the face and body by the American Board of Medical Specialties.

cold-expeller pressed oils   Oils that are extracted from vegetables without heat. Most other vegetables oils in the grocery stores, such as canola and corn oils, are heat extracted. Purchase only cold-expeller pressed vegetable oils because they don't contain trans-fatty acids. You can find them at the health food store or health food section of your grocery store.

collagen   A protein that forms the chief constituent of the connective tissues and bones. It gives skin strength and durability. Age-related declines in collagen production cause thinning of the skin, wrinkles, and sagging.

Cosmeceuticals such as vitamin C and eating foods rich in amino acids stimulate collagen production.

comedone   A pore clogged with sebum and dead skin cells.

complete protein   A food that contains all nine essential amino acids. Only animal-based foods contain complete protein.

congestion   This is skin that's bumpy and stopped up. The natural oils and skin sloughing has slowed down leaving the skin looking unclear and dull.

cortisol   An adrenal-cortex hormone. Any type of physical or mental stress induces the release of cortisol. Too much ongoing cortisol in the body causes inflammation and irritation. It's thought to be a cause of chronic disease conditions, such as diabetes, heart disease, and autoimmune disorders.

cosmeceutical   A skin care ingredient that actually alters the skin and its underlying health. Cosmeceuticals are often combined with cosmetic ingredients in skin care products.

couperose   Describes skin that has dilated or broken capillaries.

décolleté   The area in women from the base of the neck to the top of the bosom. We include this area when we talk about facial skin. The décolleté is revealed when wearing simple V-neck T-shirts, tailored blouses, and evening wear.

dioscorea   A nutrient contained in wild yam. It's not a phytoestrogen, but serves as a precursor to progesterone. The body can produce progesterone and other hormones from dioscorea.

diuretic   A food, beverage, herb, or drug that causes the body to increase the output of urine, thus drawing moisture from the cells and leaving the body with a reduced water content.

DMAE (dimethylaminoethanol)   Occurs naturally in fish. It's used for treatment of autism, dementia, mood disorders, and to improve vision. DMAE is proving beneficial in reversing the effects of skin aging, such as wrinkles and sagging. DMAE is used both topically and internally.

double-blind   A research study that uses a control group to validate a study's results. One group uses the product, one group doesn't. Neither group nor the professionals administering the study know which group is using the product or which group isn't. This is essential to truly scientific studies. Cosmetic companies typically don't follow this procedure, so their acclaimed results are not scientifically valid.

edema   An abnormal swelling of the fluid in the tissues.

elastin   A protein component of skin that helps maintain skin resilience and elasticity. When elastin is abundant and undamaged, the skin regains its shape after being folded or stretched.

electrolytes   Mineral salts that, in solution, conduct a current of electricity. Electrolytes are required by cells to regulate the flow of water molecules across cell membranes. Major electrolytes are sodium, potassium, chloride, calcium, magnesium, bicarbonate, phosphate, and sulfate.

emulsifier   A substance that helps keep oils and liquids in suspension to prevent separation of the ingredients. Without the benefits of emulsifiers, products would separate and cleaners couldn't clean your face.

enzymes   Food products or supplements that aid in digestion. Papaya contains the enzyme papain, and pineapple contains the enzyme bromelain. Both are commonly used as aids to the stomach to enhance digestion. These same enzymes, when used on the face, "digest" or break down dead skin cells and other cellular waste. They clear out the gunk and leave a brightened complexion.

exfoliants   Skin care products that break down and remove keratinized cells that naturally build up on the skin's surface. Even skin functioning at peak performance and normal skin can benefit from an exfoliant. Exfoliants help restore that healthy, translucent glow we all strive for.

extrinsic factors   These factors that affect skin are caused by the environment, your health, and how you treat your skin. For the most part, you can control the extrinsic factors that affect the condition of your skin.

food combining   Thought to be a way to eat all nine essential amino acids without eating animal products, such as by combining legumes with rice, corn, nuts, seeds, or wheat.

free radicals   Highly active chemicals in the body. They're created from many metabolic processes and also from inflammation and sun damage. They contain one or more unpaired electrons and scavenge, or steal, electrons from other molecules, thus damaging those molecules. In terms of your skin, free radicals can damage collagen and elastin.

hydroquinone   An antioxidant and skin lightener that in high concentrations is a prescription-only topical medication. Hydroquinone in low concentrations is used as an ingredient in skin care products.

immune system modulators   Foods and supplements that strengthen the immune system. They modulate the immune system so that it's neither overactive, which can lead to autoimmune diseases, nor underactive, which can lead to bacterial and viral infections.

intrinsic factors   Caused by your biological and genetic makeup. You were born with a certain type of skin and your DNA determines in part how it ages, your skin tone, and its overall plumpness and glow.

keratinization   The development of a rough quality in skin tissue. Keratin is a fiber protein in skin tissue. Keratin is made soluble with AHAs and BHAs, and can be broken down by enzyme exfoliants.

keratinized skin   When dead skin cells build up and cover up the newer skin underneath, leading to blemishes and dull skin. To remedy, use a physical exfoliant, such as cleansing grains. Use gently.

melanocytes   The cells that produce the pigment melanin. This pigment colors our skin, hair, and eyes. Melanin is heavily concentrated in skin moles.

menopause   The cessation of menstruation, occurring around the age of 50. A woman is considered to be through menopause when she hasn't had any menstrual cycles for over 12 consecutive months. The age for menopause varies, and generally ranges from about 43 through 59.

microlacerations   Miniscule or tiny tears or scrapes on the surface of the skin. Can be caused by using physical exfoliants that are too harsh, such as ground-up nutshells, buff puffs, or loofahs, and especially by using too much pressure when using physical exfoliants.

milia   Small, whitish, pear-like bumps in the skin due to retention of sebum. Another name for whiteheads.

noncomedogenic   A type of skin care product that doesn't promote the formation of blackheads and whiteheads and won't cause breakouts. Some skin care products, such as lanolin are comedogenic and can promote blackheads and breakouts.

nutrient dense   A term that refers to skin care products that contain a high concentration of added vitamins, minerals, and antioxidants. These nourish the skin and provide added protection from free radicals.

nutrient-dense foods   Contain high concentrations of vitamins, minerals, and antioxidants. They offer more nutrition per bite than other less nutrient-dense foods. An avocado is a nutrient-dense food, as is a carrot. Donuts and french fries aren't.

perimenopause   The three-to-seven-year period prior to menopause during which estrogen levels begin to drop.

photo aging   A term that refers to skin damage from the sun.

phytoestrogens   Estrogenlike compounds found in foods. When you eat these foods, they act like the estrogens produced in the body. Phytoestrogens are weaker than the estrogen your body produces. Estrogen helps keep your skin thicker with higher levels of elastin and collagen.

sebum   The semifluid secretion of the sebaceous glands, consisting chiefly of fat, keratin, and cellular material.

silicone derivatives   Ingredients in moisturizers that sit on the surface of the skin and lock in moisture without clogging pores and causing breakouts. They also give the skin a soft and smooth texture.

skin care line   A term that refers to a brand's skin care products. This is a common usage in the skin care industry and at department store sales counters.

slip   The sensation that the skin is smooth and ever so slightly slippery. Slip lets you apply foundation easily, allowing it to glide on smoothly and evenly. You have a healthy amount of slip when you touch your skin and your hand easily glides over the surface without catching on rough or dry patches.

SPF (Sun Protection Factor)   All sunscreens are currently labeled with an SPF that lets you know how long you can stay in the sun before burning. Wear a sunscreen with an SPF of 15 or more to get adequate sun protection.

spritz   To spray the toner on your face. Hold the atomizer or spray bottle about 12 to 14 inches from your face, close your eyes, and spritz your face two or three times. Feels refreshing and cooling.

stye   An inflammation of one of the sebaceous glands of the eyelid.

synergistically   The combined interaction of the three products—cleanser, toner, and moisturizer—is greater than the sum of their effects individually.

telangiectasia   The chronic dilation of groups of capillaries that causes elevated dark red blotches on the skin.

vagus nerve   Also known as the wandering nerve. It originates in the brain and runs along the front of the neck, then down into the esophagus, heart, and stomach. Important for swallowing, digestion, hearing, and heart function, dysfunction of the vagus nerve can result in ringing in the ears, heart palpitations, heartburn, and acid reflux.

Index

vitamins, 85
    acne, 124
    as cosmeceuticals, 85-86
vitiligo, 184

W–X–Y–Z

wandering nerve, 269
warts, 184
washing. *See* cleansing
water, 204
    dehydration, 205
    drinking, 205-207
    excessive, 209-210
    purified, 208
    taste, 207
waterproof sunscreens, 174
waxing, 60-62
websites
    AAAASF, 304
    body rolling, 228
    glycemic index, 217
    GlycoLoad, 218
    Light Boxes, 172
    Maxi-Backsie, 228
    psoriasis, 164
whiteheads, 133

Xs (exercise), 269

zinc, 124

Check Out These
Best-Selling
COMPLETE IDIOT'S GUIDES®

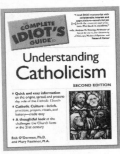

Understanding Catholicism
SECOND EDITION

1-59257-085-2
$18.95

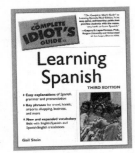

Learning Spanish
THIRD EDITION

0-02-864451-4
$18.95

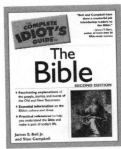

The Bible
SECOND EDITION

0-02-864382-8
$18.95

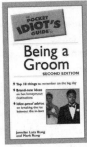

Being a Groom
SECOND EDITION

0-02-864456-5
$9.95

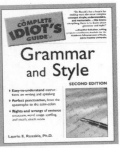

Grammar and Style
SECOND EDITION

1-59257-115-8
$16.95

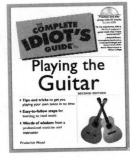

Playing the Guitar
SECOND EDITION

0-02-864244-9
$21.95 w/CD

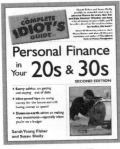

Personal Finance in Your 20s & 30s
SECOND EDITION

0-02-864374-7
$19.95

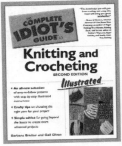

Knitting and Crocheting
SECOND EDITION
Illustrated

1-59257-089-5
$16.95

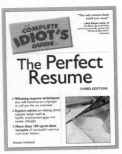

The Perfect Resume
THIRD EDITION

0-02-864440-9
$14.95

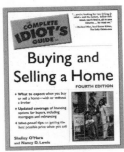

Buying and Selling a Home
FOURTH EDITION

1-59257-120-4
$18.95

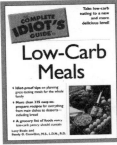

Low-Carb Meals

1-59257-180-8
$18.95

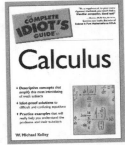

Calculus

0-02-864365-8
$18.95

More than 450 titles in 30 different categories
Available at booksellers everywhere

ALPHA